KETO AIR FRYER COOKBOOK FOR BEGINNERS

1001 RECIPES TO HELP YOU LOSE WEIGHT FAST AND EASY

By

Beverly Laila Wilson

attempt has been made to provide accurate, up to date and reliable complete information. No warranties of any kind are expressed or implied. Readers acknowledge that the author is not engaging in the rendering of legal, financial, medical or professional advice. The content of this book has been derived from various sources. Please consult a licensed professional before attempting any techniques outlined in this book.

By reading this document, the reader agrees that under no circumstances are is the author responsible for any losses, direct or indirect, which are incurred as a result of the use of the information contained within this document, including, but not limited to, errors, omissions, or inaccuracies.

Table of Contents

1 Introduction

You can only dream of a world in which onions rings, chicken pieces, and crispy fries have the same taste and are healthier. To some extent, unbelievable, but the air makes it feasible. The machine uses a small amount of oil and warm air to cook and delicately crisp the meal. On the contrary, conventional deep frying requires that the food be dipped into approximately three cups of oil. Larger amounts of oil production more considerable quantities of fat than roasting or baking.

Most air fryers only require a tablespoon of oil, nevertheless. If you are interested in this device, possessing an Air fryer is like getting a savior plus with tasty recipes, this wonderful gadget can be explored, folks! The shortage of oil does not translate into food without any texture or taste. One research contrasts deep-fried French fries with air-fried and shows the resemblance in moisture, color, and texture - yet fat content differ. As a result, less fat leads to fewer calories, so cooking with an air fryer can indirectly help with weight loss rather than deep frying. Many people are decreasing their calorie intake using air fryers by an average of 70–80%, as reported at Cleveland Clinic, Ohio.

Some research also indicates the production of dangerous compounds, such as carcinogenic acrylamide in air-fryer cooking is limited. This is seen in foods that contain high amounts of carbohydrates, which cook by means of heat-intensive methods, such as frying.

Well, traditional deep-frying, study shows that air-frying will minimize acrylamide by 90%. Be cautious not to overcook the food in an air fryer as blackened foods can also be carcinogenic. Taking into account these benefits be aware that air frying is still technically frying and cannot substitute other cooking methods quite accurately. A noticeable concern is over-the-air cooking or replenishing balanced cooking practices with some frying, such as baking, steaming or grilling.

It can have a detrimental effect on diet and calorie consumption. Ensure sure you don't waste your kitchen equipment, fireplaces, and other kitchens. The important point is that air frying is a great procedure that helps us to eat fried food without extra concentrations of oil and fat from deep frying.

The air fryer is here to greatly benefit you. Keep in mind; this is not an exact substitution for other healthier ways of cooking. If you want more opportunities to best your own cooking time, immerse yourself in this book to learn some astonishingly tasty recipes.

2   What Is An Air Fryer?

An air fryer is a modern kitchen gadget that cooks food using extremely hot air instead of oil. This provides a low-fat variant of food usually served in a deep frying pan. As a result, often fatty foods, such as French-fried foods, fried chicken and onion rings, are made without oil or with a fat level of up to 80 percent lower than conventional cooking techniques. The Air fryer offers healthy fried foods and meals that help you to get rid of calories that come from fried food while also providing you the pain, taste, and consistency that you like.

This household device works consistently and efficiently by rotating extremely hot air around a food product in a closed space. The sun makes the food product crooked and dry on the surface, but inside it is smooth and moist. The air fryer can be used on almost anything. You will barbecue, bake and roast in addition to frying. Due to its varied cooking choices, it is easier to prepare every form of meal every day.

2.1 Why Use It

Low-Fat Meals: The biggest advantage of the air fryer, obviously, is the hot-air ventilation used to cook food ingredients from all directions, removing the need to use gasoline. It helps those on a low-fat diet to cook delightfully balanced meals easily.

Healthier Foods& Environment: Air fryers are designed for the processing of nutritious foods with up to 80% reduced-fat without fattening oils. It makes it possible to shed weight because you can afford to consume the processed food while retaining calories and saturated fat. It is easier to turn to a healthy life while using this machine. Your home often gets rid of the smell of deep-fried foods, which often linger in the house even after many hours of deep-frying.

Multipurpose Use: The air fryer makes it easier for you to multitask as you can cook several foods concurrently. Your all-in-one gadget will barbecue, bake, fry and roast the meals you love! You don't require multiple gadgets for different tasks. This is highly probable to do other tasks with different devices. This will barbecue beef, roast vegetables and bake pastries. This is an easy substitute for your microwave, deep fryer, and grill.

Extremely Safe: Recall how cautious you will be when you load a deep fryer with chicken or any other ingredients? You want to prevent the hot oil from leaking and frying your skin because it is still really dry. You don't have to think about the bulk skin caused by hot oil spillage on your air fryer. It fries anything and is completely free. Nevertheless, use cooking gloves when moving the fryer to prevent fire hazards. Hold your air fryer out of sight of children.

Easy Clean Up: The air fryer does not leave any grease, therefore, no residue. Clean-up periods are enjoyable as there are no oils spilled onto walls and surfaces, and there are no plans to scrap or scrub. It's not important to waste time making sure everything is squeaky clean. The parts of the air fryer are constructed from a non-stick material that keeps food from sticking to surfaces, making it difficult to clean. These parts can be washed and maintained easily. They are reusable and dishwasher-safe also.

Save Valuable Time: Tight schedules encourage people to make tasty meals using the quickness of the air fryer. In less than 15 minutes, for example, you can make French frieze and bake a cake in 25 minutes.

You may also enjoy crispy golden fries or chicken tenders within a few minutes. The air fryer is just the right option if you're still on the go because you will waste less time in the kitchen. It helps you to handle your stressful working life and make your day more productive.

2.2   What Can't You Make?

You can't make a fluid mixture, such as this battered Crispy Beer Fish. You cannot do something in huge quantities too, so be ready for batch cooking if you intend on inviting people over.

Cost: Air fryers cost anywhere between $100 and $300, on the pricey side of home equipment, based on their size and highlights. Identify the best air fryer for your culture and values.

Space: The air fryer is definitely no small tool; it is more extensive than a toaster. You must offer considerable storage (or counter) room to one building.

Aptitudes: Air fryers are essentially appropriate and play. Specify the time and the temperature in the bottle and the bam!

Taste and Surface: While an air fryer will yield results much closer to deep browning than your griddle can, it is still not the same by the end of the day.

It is more advantageous: it can be claimed that by using less oil it creates more valuable fuel. Frozen fried fries in an air frying pan produce 4 and 6 grams of fat in some cases, relative to their deep-frozen fried counterpart in an incredible 17 grams in each serving.

2.3   What Should I Look For In An Air Fryer?

A single brand like Instant Pot does not dominate air fryer sales as opposed to pressure cookers. When you're on the market for the right air fryer for you, there are certain features that should be considered.

Loading. Many models come fitted with front drawers to load, unload, and some have a flip-top cover. The experts recommend comfort and health drawer typestyles.

Ease of use. Are the control systems easy to comprehend and run? Perhaps you want everybody in your home to be able to utilize the air-fryer. A few people read the manual - everyone else wants to go up and wing it. Even the basket should be easy to empty and clean.

Controls. While certain models are set up to 400 degrees, others have only one setting for temperatures. Most would want to have a leftover reheat press as well as presets for meals, such as fish and chicken.

Functionality can make a difference. Could you break cooking to turn your meal or to stir it? You will reset the temperature and time of certain devices.

Size. For one or two individuals, the majority of countertop versions are wide enough. If you are cooking for more than one batch, you will possibly have to purchase a larger model with lots of space. You should buy a smaller model. Many versions have a toaster and an air fryer, meaning that some energy can be saved if your toaster oven is replaced.

Tips For Better Air Frying

Pat foods dry. Bring everything you like crispy and browned, like beef, fish, and vegetables, before frying in the oven.

Avoid overfilling the basket. An air freezer depends on a fan to blow hot air efficiently to cook food. Crowding your basket will stop hot air touching all the ingredients, which will slow down your cooking to give you poor and soggy results. Many versions have full lines and the manual will also provide instructions. Our experts typically claim that they will not fill the basket more than 3/2 if the maximum fill line on the basket is not labelled.

Check food often. You cannot turn on the lamp and monitor the status of food through the window, like cooking food in the oven. You cannot see the ingredients when you cook with an air fryer – they're hidden away in a drawer-style basket, which makes it very difficult to grasp how this is achieved. The cooking times will differ dramatically from one worker to another. Check the food every so often during the cooking process to prevent overcooking. In some versions, this is as easy as removing your cabinet, but on others, it may be appropriate to take a pause before you prepare.

Flip the food as it cooks. Using thongs or shake the bowl for even results during the cooking.

Experiment with homemade favorites. The shop-bought fries look fine, but an air fryer helps the actual work: cut potatoes into standard bits for crispy French fries and boil them for 30 minutes in water. After which you can drain, rinse, dry, and coat delicately with oil before even air frying.

Including two workers who have checked food recipes since joining CR, people who like to eat and make that also find that they improved along the way. Be mindful that cooking time and temperature differ according to the type of air fryer you have.

2.4   Tips For Usage

Shake It: Be sure to open the air fryer and push cooking items quickly as they "Fry" in the jar of the machine - littler items like French fries and chips will stack. Pivot/turn these items every 5-10 minutes for the best results.

Try Not To Stuff: Give plenty of space to cooking objects with the intention that the air can run viably; that's what gives you fresh results. Cook in parts and small bunches on the air fryer.

Ace Other Cooking Strategies: The air fryer is not only for slow cooking; it's also exceptional for other strong cooking methods, such as baking, broiling, and flame broiling. You should even try cooking salmon in it!

Keep It Dry: Pat dry foods, particularly marinated foods, before cooking. Doing so would prevent unnecessary smoke and spraying. Foods with a high fat composition like chicken wings and breasts typically deposit fat while cooking. And make sure that you drain the stored fat from the air fryer's bottom once in a while.

Space Your Foods: Congestion in the air fryer is a no-no. Give it plenty of space if you want your food to cook properly so that air can distribute well. You want to enjoy your meals fresh, right? Overcrowding restricts the passage of air over the food. So make sure foods are spread out.

Spray Foods: If using your air fryer, you'll need your cooking spray because it helps to avoid foods from sticking to the pan. Slather foods gently or only apply a little bit of oil.

Cook In Batches: The air fryer has only a small cooking space. If you're cooking for a large number of people, you'll need to cook them in batches.

Shower Cooking Objects: Delicately shower items with cooking spray or add a tad of oil to make sure they don't stick to the crate.

Preheat air fryer if it has not been in service for some time. Heat it up for up to 3-5 minutes to enable proper heat-up.

Now you can use your air fryer to prepare the nutritious and savory recipes carefully picked below. Only follow the directions and you and your family will enjoy well-balanced meals.

3 Is Air-Frying As Healthy As You Think?

Can An Air fryer Help Cut Fat Content?

Deep-fried foods are often higher in fat than those, which are prepared using other cooking techniques. For example, a fried chicken breast contains more fat than the equivalent cooked chicken amount. A few producers promise that using an air fryer will remove up to a large number of the excess material of fried nourishments. This is because air fryers basically need less fat than traditional deep fryers. Although there are various plans for deep-fried dishes that can require up to 3 cups of oil, air-fried foods can need only about one tablespoon.

It means that deep fryers use something like several times more oil than air fryers and while the nourishment absorbs not all of that oil, using an air fryer will remove the food's general fat content entirely. One review examined the characteristics of deep-fried and air-fried French fries and found that air-searing brought about a final item with considerably less fat and a comparable quality of shading and dampness. This can have a big effect on your wellbeing, as a higher fat intake from vegetable oils has been associated with an increased risk of conditions, such as cardiovascular disease and irritation.

Switching To An Air Fryer May Possibly Aid In Weight Loss

Deep-fried foods are not only higher in fat, but are also higher in calories at the same time and can increase the weight gain. In a study of 33,542 Spanish people, higher acceptance of fried food has been correlated with greater danger. When you plan to trim your waistline, it might be a good place to exchange your deep-fried nutrients for air-fried food. Eating fats contain more than twice as much as separate macronutrients including protein and sugars in nine calories per gram of fat.

Since the fat content of air-fried foods is smaller than that of deep-fried foods, it may be an easy way to save calories and lose weight.

Air Fryers Can Decrease The Formation Of Harmful Compounds

While being higher in fat and calories, frying food can also create potentially harmful compounds, such as acrylamide.

Acrylamide is a compound produced during high-heat cooking methods, such as frying in carbohydrate-rich foods. Acrylamide is listed as a "Probable Carcinogen," according to the International Agency for Research on Cancer, indicating that some research shows that acrylamide may be related to cancer growth.

While the findings are conflicting, some studies have found a correlation between dietary acrylamide and increased risk of cancer of the kidney, endometrial, and ovary. Air-frying your food can help lower the acrylamide content of your fried foods, rather than using a deep fryer.

In addition, one study found that, compared with conventional deep-frying, air-frying reduced acrylamide by 90%. It is important to remember, however, that more harmful compounds that still be produced during the air-frying process.

Aldehydes, heterocyclic amines, and polycyclic aromatic hydrocarbons are all other potentially hazardous chemicals produced by high-heat cooking and may be linked with higher cancer risk. More work is required to evaluate how the formation of these compounds can impact air-frying.

Air-Frying May Be Healthier Than Deep-Frying

Air-fried foods can be safer in many ways than deep-fried foods. These are lower in fat, calories and even certain potentially harmful compounds found in common fried foods. If you are looking to lose weight or lower your fat intake without altering or removing fried foods, it may be a good choice to turn to an air fryer. Keep in mind, however, that just because it may be a better option than deep-frying doesn't mean it's a perfect option in terms of your overall health.

While air-fried foods may be more nutritious than deep-fried foods, it's essential to note that when frying with oil they are nearly identical to fried food. A host of studies have shown that consuming fried foods can be associated with various adverse health effects. A survey of 15,362 men, for instance, showed that consuming more fried food was associated with a greater risk of heart failure.

Recent work has shown that eating deep-fried foods regularly can be associated with increased risk of certain types of cancer, including prostate, lung, and oral cancers. Many conditions, such as type 2 diabetes and high blood pressure have often been linked with consuming fried foods.

While research specifically on the effects of air-fried foods is minimal, reducing your consumption of all fried foods is advised to help promote better health. Alternatively, use safer methods of cooking, such as baking, roasting, steaming or sautéing to improve flavor and prevent the negative effects of fried foods on the skin.

Using an air fryer will decrease the amount of fat, calories and possibly hazardous compounds in your food compared with deep-frying. Nonetheless, air-fried foods are similar to conventionally fried foods that can be associated with adverse health conditions while frying with oil and consuming them regularly. While air fryers might be a better alternative to deep fryers, the best option when it comes to your health is to reduce your consumption of fried foods altogether.

4 What Is Ketogenic Diet?

It's a high fat, low carb diet that can transform your body into a fat-burning device. The diet of the keto is brief for a ketogenic diet. Ketogenic diets provide an appropriate diet of protein intake, an elevated level of fat and a small intake of carbohydrates. It was developed in the first place as a unique diet to control the signs of epilepsy in children. Daily meals give sufficient protein to ensure growth and repair under this diet. The calories are measured and provided in enough quantities to maintain the right weight and height for the child.

The keto diet transforms how your body metabolizes food into energy. Naturally, your body transforms carbohydrates (imagine pasta and bread) into energy glucose. Eating lots of fat and few carbs bring you in ketosis, a metabolic condition where your body releases fat rather than carbs for fuel.

4.1 How Does Diet Work?

The ketogenic diet pushes the body into a stage of ketosis. The body tends primarily to use carbohydrates as energy sources. The reason is that carbohydrates can be easily digested and absorbed. When the body is without carbohydrates, fats and proteins are used. Essentially, the body hierarchically uses energy. First, while it is available, the body uses carbohydrates. As a next alternative source, the body moves into fats. The last stage, usually in extreme deprivation of carbohydrates and fatty stores, is protein conversion into energy. The digestion of proteins leads to loss of muscle, as the body digests the muscle proteins.

Generally, the body enters a process of ketosis. It takes place during the fasting period. One example of this is during sleep. When the body rebuilds and expands through sleep it continues to burn fats for energy.

Carbohydrates constitute most calories in an ordinary average meal. The body carbohydrates are used as energy and other nutrients (i.e., fats and proteins) are stored Many calories in the ketogenic diet are composed of fats instead of carbohydrates. In a ketogenic diet, carbohydrate is very small and is used instantly. There is an obvious energy deficit due to the low intake of carbohydrates. The body turns to the fats it has accumulated. This switches to a fat burner from a carbohydrate user. The fats in the recently devoured meal are not instantly used; instead, they are saved for the next round. The fats of the recent meal are used as energy sources for fat-burning, and some are left to be preserved. Therefore, in order to provide the immediate energy required, the Ketogenic diet must have a high fat intake and still have a portion of the stock. Stored fat is extremely important so that the body does not absorb the protein in the muscles at fasting times.

In addition, these cycles are common in a series of days. Fasting periods occur in between meals and sleep. During these times the body also needs a constant energy supply. Protein in the muscles is next in line as the source of energy if no stored fat is present. Your diet needs to be high in fat in order to prevent this

Ketogenic diets are mainly designed to imitate starvation mode. This decreases calories and significantly eliminates carbohydrates, thus depriving the body of carbohydrates instantly and quickly converted. This compels the body to shift to the mode which consumes fat. It also induces the secretion of catecholamines (fat mobilizing hormones), cortisol (break-down and metabolic hormones) and growth hormones. This triad of hormones triggers the state of ketosis or a fat burn.

5 Ketogenic Diet Health Benefits

Ketogenic diets have similar benefits to those of other low-carb and high-fat diets, which tend to be better than traditional low-carb diets. View keto as an extra packed low-carb diet that maximizes benefits. On the other hand, it can be more difficult to do as well and the risk of side effects can be raised a little.

Weight Loss - Turning the body to a machine for fat burning will help to reduce weight. Fat burns are increased significantly while insulin–the hormone that stores fat–decreases considerably. This seems to make the lack of weight without appetite much better. By contrast with other foods, low-carb diets and keto diets lead to more successful weight loss according to 30 high-quality scientific studies. Among conventional diets, the Ketogenic diet has found a niche. It now comes under many diets due to its reported adverse effect in weight loss promotion. First, several eyebrows were raised to the idea of losing weight through a high-fat diet. Ketogenic dieting is now slowly taken into account as part of weight loss programs over time and with better results. The weight gain in carbs is higher than in fats. Note the hormone insulin improves carbohydrate accumulation, thereby gaining weight. Removing and sustaining a minimal consumption of carbohydrates may cause a significant decrease in weight over time.

Reduces Inflammation - Inflammation is the natural reaction of your body to an invader that it is considered harmful. Too much inflammation is terrible news because the risk of chronic diseases increases. A keto-diet will decrease inflammation in the body when inflammatory pathways are shut off and free radicals are lower than glucose

Appetite Control - You would definitely have new control of your appetite in a keto diet. Since your body burns fat 24/7, you have constant access to saved energy for weeks or months that greatly reduces hunger feelings. This is a very common occurrence that is confirmed by research. This makes eating less difficult and losing excess weight easier; wait until you're tired before feeding. It also simplifies intermittent fasting, something, which can overcome type 2 diabetes and promote weight loss over and above the influence of keto only. Additionally, by not having to snack all the time, you might save tons of money and time. Some people feel they just have to eat on a keto diet twice daily, and some once per day. Difficulty to tackle hunger can theoretically also assist with conditions, such as sugar and food addiction. Ultimately, it can be part of the solution where you feel satisfied. Food could avoid being an enemy and become your partner, or just fuel whatever you like.

Control Blood Sugar And Reverse Type 2 Diabetes - Studies show that a ketogenic diet is good for controlling type 2 diabetes and sometimes even curing the condition entirely. That makes complete sense as Keto decreases blood sugar levels, eliminates the need for drugs and lowers the potentially negative effects of high levels of insulin. Assuming that a keto diet can cure current diabetes type 2, treatment and reversal of pre-diabetes are likely to be effective.

Improved Health Markers - Numerous studies indicate that low-carb diets boost many essential heart disease risk factors, such as the cholesterol profile, with a moderate effect on total cholesterol and LDL levels. Increased blood sugar, glucose, and blood pressure are also common. The frequently improved markers are correlated with something termed "Metabolic Syndrome," weight improvements, type 2 diabetes reversal, waist circumference and much more.

Energy And Mental Performance - Many people specifically use ketogenic diets to enhance mental performance. It is also common for people in ketosis to feel an energy boost. The brain needs no dietary carbs when on Keto. It is powered by Ketones 24-7, an efficient fuel for the brain Ketosis thus leads to continuous fuel flow into the brain, therefore, it prevents issues with large blood sugar fluctuations. This can lead to better focus, relaxation, brain fog resolution and improved clarity of mind.

A Calmer Stomach - A keto diet can lead to calmer belly, less nausea, fewer cramps, and discomfort, also leading to better treatment of IBS. This is a great advantage for some people and it takes usually only a day or two to feel it.

Increased Physical Endurance - In theory ketogenic diets can improve your physical endurance by increasing your exposure to the huge energy reserves of your fat stores. The body only needs a few hours of intense training or less for the availability of processed carbohydrates. Nonetheless, the fat stores have sufficient energy to last for months. Furthermore, the decrease in the body fat percentage, which can be obtained with a keto diet, is another potential benefit. For different competitive sports, including endurance sports, the decrease in body fat weight may be appreciated.

Keto Diets And Epilepsy - The ketogenic diet is an established and often successful epilepsy treatment since the 1920s. Traditionally mostly used for children, adults have also benefited from it in recent years. Using an epilepsy ketogenic diet may make certain individuals take less or no anti-epileptic medicine while they may be seizure-free. This could reduce the side effects of drugs and thus increase cognitive performance.

Keto Diets And Cancer - Ongoing research suggests that the ketogenic diet can contribute to the relief of cancer. Basically, it "Starves Cancer" to suppress the symptoms.

Keto Diets And Alzheimer Disease - Research shows that when an Alzheimer's patient is on a ketogenic diet, it increases the memory function. Some of their memory and thought processes are restored.

Keto Diets And Neurological Disorders - ALS and Parkinson's disease are some of the neurological conditions benefiting from the ketogenic diet. The diet supports mitochondrial affected nerves. The signs are thus intensified.

Gluten Allergy - Most may have a gluten allergy that is not diagnosed. After a ketogenic diet, conditions, such as bloating and gastrointestinal pain improved. In most carbohydrate foods, gluten is high. Gluten consumption is also kept to a very minimum by removing a wide range of carbohydrates in the diet. The symptoms of gluten are thus eliminated as well.

May Increase Lifespan - Ketosis activates pathways to prolong your lifespan. Good gene expression is one of these. Ketosis activates genes that counter oxidative stress and control survival metabolism. The other is a defense against mitochondria. Some antioxidants are produced in your mitochondria when producing ketones like BHB, and harmful oxidants are removed to keep your cells from becoming sick. It means that keto causes a powerful antioxidant reaction that clearly does not happen with glucose.

Unlocks Metabolic Flexibility - The ketogenic diet is not the regular diet for loss of weight because it modifies everything important in your body. Your cells use glucose for energy like almost every other diet. In keto, glucose is substituted by ketones as the primary source of energy. This switch stimulates the ability to change between fats and carbs if necessary to make optimal use of both. For example, an individual who adapts to keto can go on holiday and have carbohydrate meals for a few days, and then turn over in a day or less to ketosis via carbohydrates and fasting. This metabolic versatility is typical in your hunter-gatherer ancestors who changed continuously from fasting to feeding, based on food availability (where the body is working on ketones). Ketosis effectively preserves the developed body's metabolic versatility, which prevents you from obesity and diabetes.

6 Keto Side Effects And What To Do About Them

A ketogenic diet is usually perfectly safe for many, but there are a few side effects:

Dehydration And Muscle Cramps - Carbs need water to be stored Fat doesn't seem to. On a keto diet, you retain less liquid, and instead of keeping salt, the kidneys constantly remove sodium. Therefore, it is simple, especially in the first few weeks, to dehydrate the food keto. Your muscles can also begin to cramp with fatigue and low electrolytes.

Do this: Focus on the body's three primary electrolytes on magnesium, sodium, and potassium, and ensure that you drink extra water. This is especially important when you're working on keto. Hydration also helps prevent keto flu symptoms.

Decreased Metabolic Flexibility - Several people report that they struggle to handle carbohydrates while eating a strict keto diet in the long term and that makes perfect sense. If you don't eat carbs at all, you don't have to control your insulin receptors. It's like keeping the lights on throughout the day —waste of energy.

After you've been intense keto for a long time, the body seems to reduce the production of insulin (the hormone which causes the cells to use carbohydrates as fuel). Many parts of your body depend on glucose, such as the brain's glial cells, which perform repair and immune function. You won't run at full capacity if your body cells are good at using fat for fuel and horrible at using carbohydrates.

Do this: Experiment one day a week with carbs by eating 150 grams of high-quality carbs.

Insomnia - There's no study on keto and sleep disorders, but there are some who claim that keto meal keeps them up at midnight. You would likely better be able to eat some high-quality carbohydrates at night when you notice you have trouble sleeping on the keto. Such problems are common on strict keto and form a large part of why the bulletproof diet requires quality carbohydrates.

Do this: Take one raw honey tablespoon before sleep.

Not Enough Fiber - It can be tough to get enough food when you consume less than 20 grams of carbs a day. Low consumption of fiber may lead to constipation, an increased risk of colon cancer and Irritable Bowel Syndrome (IBS).

Do this:

- Choose leafy, bright, fiber-rich foods to deliver the rest of your keto carbs.
- Try to eat more fiber-rich foods, such as sweet potatoes and butternut squash in a cyclical keto diet.
- Consider a prebiotic fiber that feeds beneficial intestinal bacteria like bulletproof InnenFuel.
- Make sure you get 2 to 2.5 teaspoons of salt per day to ensure that your bowels are kept consistently insufficient water.
- Keep hydrated and stack on magnesium and potassium–you can find essential electrolytes in avocado, spinach, and other supplements.
- Maintain a diary for food. Follow up what you eat and remember to take not on foods that do and do not digest well.
- Exercise will allow you to manage your digestive system properly and sustain it.

Diarrhea - Many people experience diarrhea at the opposite end of the spectrum, particularly if they're not used to a higher fat diet.

Do this:

- Start with MCT oils at a slow pace: MCT oil is a fatty acid that easily energizes the body into ketones. It contributes to fueling your body, particularly when it adapts to keto. Your digestive system may take a bit of time to get used to MCT oils. Begin with 1 tsp and work up from there.

- A digestive enzyme can be added: If your body is finding it difficult to properly digest fats, consider lipase, a fat digestive enzyme or hydrochloric acid that helps increase the amount of stomach acid and promote digestion in the body.

Keto Rash - A change in diet can induce itchy, red rash on your back, head, neck, and axis for a very small number of people who try keto. Keto rash, also regarded as Prurigo pigmentosa, is not life-threatening or harmful. The precise reasons are still not known, although scientists point to variations in hormones, intestinal microbes and exposure to pathogens as possible causes.

Do this: Consult your doctor and use the following methods to treat keto rash:

- Reintroduce some healthy carbs: You do not have to completely go on bread-binge, but you may want to add good, high-quality carbs, such as yams, carrots, butternut squash, pumpkin, sweet potatoes when you suddenly switch into keto diets.

- Try to prevent irritants: Keto rash can intensify with rubbing, sweat or cold, just as most rashes. Do not intensify the irritated skin by wearing loose, aerobic clothes or avoiding fragrances or sweat activity until the skin is clean.

- Support the skin: This helps you increase your healing time and relax the rash by offering anti-inflammatory foods and supplements. Try to add foods, such as this turmeric latte, a DHA omega-3 supplement, or those top 5 healthy skin nutrients.

Keto Flu - Keto flu is a normal response that your body experiences when it changes its energy from burning sugar to fat. Keto flu, also called carb withdrawal, typically occurs between 24 to 48 hours. Symptoms include migraine, irritability, brain fog, muscular pain, insomnia, poor concentration, and sugar appetite.

Many people are more affected by the keto flu than others. You will experience mild symptoms only if you eat a diet low in refined sugar and starch before you go into Keto.

You may have more symptoms of abstinence, particularly glucose, with a high sugar and carbohydrates diet.

How does the keto flu come about? Your body needs to learn to exhaust its backup supply of energy while restricting carbohydrates, and to do so three major changes must take place:

- Sodium and water flush: when you ingest fewer carbohydrates, the level of insulin will reduce and the kidney will be alerted to release sodium from the bloodstream. The water removes sodium from your body, causing a reduction to about 10 pounds of water weight. Generally, all this happens in the first five days. Dizziness, vomiting, muscle cramping, fatigue, and digestive problems are the result of glycogen deficiency and low insulin levels Do your part at this stage to drink plenty of water and electrolytes - these cell symptoms will ease.

- T3 levels of thyroid hormones can decline: T3 is a thyroid gland-produced hormone. Dietary and thyroid functions are intimately linked so that the T3 levels can decrease when you cut carbohydrates. Both hormones control body temperature, appetite, and heart rate in tandem with T4, another thyroid hormone. If your body falls for a ketogenic diet, the lower levels of hormones will keep you fogged and exhausted.

- Increased levels of cortisol: T3 change in hormones is closely linked to a fourth hormonal switch-increased level of cortisol. The body is told by a ketogenic diet that you're starving. To order to increase energy levels in a carb-restricted diet, the body allows stress hormones, such as cortisol, to be released. This is an indication that your amount of cortisol has sprung up when you suffer irritability and insomnia. Don't worry: the level of cortisol will collapse to their old levels when you adapt to use fat and ketones as a new fuel.

Do this: To beat the keto flu, try these remedies.

- Keep hydrated. Use your current body weight and break it by two to calculate the total amount of water you need. How many ounces do you have to have? For starters, you can reach for 70 ounces of water every day if you actually measure close 140 pounds. Bone broth adds a part of water to your diet and an intake of electrolytes (sodium and potassium) to relieve your cellular pain.

- Electrolyte replacement. Replenish the electrolytes is an ideal way to feel better quickly. Note: potassium, magnesium and sodium, the main stars. If your diet doesn't give you plenty, which can be hard to achieve on low carbon, add it as a supplement.

- Feed fatter, MCTs in general. You can speed up your adaptation process by increasing your fat consumption. A warning: the bulk of fats must go to the lungs, muscles and fat cells through your lymphatic system before they enter the liver. These can only be converted into ketones to be used as energy by the body. MCT oil is unique because it goes directly to the liver-just as sugars-after ingestion, so it can be used instantly.

- Have a good rest. Get good rest. A good sleeping night is a very good thing in the capture of keto control. This controls the levels of cortisol, which will potentially lessen the effects of your flu. Set 7-9 hours a night.

- Meditate and exercise (moderate). The second word is noticeable: moderate. Yeah, yeah. The purpose here is to reduce (especially first) cortisol levels, so anything that alleviates pressure should help. The key can be Yoga and light runs. Try to meditate if exercising isn't yours. In the end, probably the best thing is to stay in the fitness center before you change your diet.

- Take powdered charcoal. Activated charcoal detoxifies the skin by dumping fat into your bloodstream. Charcoal binds to chemical substances whose particles, including several toxic molds, BPA and pesticide, have positive charges.

- Take a supplement of the exogenous ketone. Exogenous ketones allow you to increase relaxation and strength by increasing your blood ketone levels. Remember that they aren't a substitute for an appropriate keto diet, but they might help you get it - especially on flu. When you choose to go along this path, try to spread the first three to five days of keto flu with smaller doses of the drug.

If everything else goes wrong, up the intake of your carb Increasing fat just does not reduce keto flu symptoms for some individuals. If this is the case and by adding more fat you have reached your boundaries and still have flu-like symptoms, your carb consumption should be increased just a little more.

7 What To Eat On Keto

The diet in keto is quite straightforward: mainly eat healthy fats (75% of your day to day calories), some protein (about 20%), and very little carbohydrates (about 5%). That combination puts you into ketosis.

Choose the low-carb foods you want, including beef, fish, dairy, vegetables and good fats. Consult this comprehensive list of foods and check these recipes for food ideas. Many people eat 30-150 grams of net carbohydrates per day more.

Net carbs mean that fibers and sugar alcohol (such as xylitol) may be subtracted from your daily carb count - as they do not affect your blood sugar or stored as glycogen, a form of glucose storage.

Types Of Keto Diets

Standard Keto: Every day, you eat a very low carb diet (less than 50 grams net carbs per day). Many followers of keto eat only about 20 grams a day.

Cyclical Keto: Eat high fat and very low carbohydrates food for 5 to 6 days a week (less than 50 g of net carbohydrate daily). Take a carb refeed-day (about 150 grams) on day 7. Another category includes the Bulletproof Diet, but it increases its quality even more efficiently, with irregular levels, protein fasting and a focus on low inflammatory, nutrient-rich goods.

Targeted Keto: You follow the standard Keto diet, but consume added carbohydrates 30 minutes to an hour before the intensive training. Glucose aims to improve efficiency, and after learning you can return to ketosis. This kind of food can work for you if your energy fails in the gym.

Dirty Keto: Dirty Keto follows the same fat, protein and glucose ratio as a regular keto diet, but it is with a twist: wherever those macronutrients are derived is not important. Dinner might be the Diet Pepsi or bunless Big Mac.

Moderate Keto: Eat high fat every day with a net carb of 100-150 grams. Women are often better at using this diet—carbohydrates that impair their hormone activity may sometimes get messy. Many participants also note that on training days, they run out less than 100 grams of carbs.

Protein in a ketogenic diet primarily contains three important types of food. A vegetable or fruit, a food rich in protein and fat source.

Fats - Ketogenic diet needs more dietary fat. These can be used in the cooking process, such as frying and grilling. Often, sauces and dressings that take on the shape of fats. Top a piece of butter steak is also a way of adding fats to your diet. Ketogenic fats are the safest kind of fats. The best ones, like MCTs and coconut oil, are medium-chain triglycerides. The fats are metabolized rapidly to create ketones.

Other good fats for ketosis are:

- High oleic - Safflower oils, Sunflower oils
- Omega-3 and Omega-6 fatty acids – Trout, Salmon, Tuna, Shellfish
- Monounsaturated and Saturated fats - Olive oil, Red palm oil, Butter, Cheese, Avocado, Egg yolks
- Non-hydrogenated oils (when cooking) - Beef tallow, Non-hydrogenated lards, Coconut oil
- Other fat sources - Peanut butter, Chicken skin, Fat on meats, Coconut butter

Proteins - In a ketogenic diet, every form of meat is practically allowed. The type of cut and preparation is not differentiated, e.g., Pork, Beef, Veal, Venison, Lamb

Poultry is of any sort, too. It is best to have your skin on because it increases your food's fat content. Breading and batter should not be included in the preparation because they have high levels of carbohydrate Acceptable arrangements depend on the desires of individuals, e.g., Chicken, Quail, Turkey, and Duck

Seafood is also a good source of protein. Some have high fatty acids, vitamins and minerals omega-3, which can lead to sustaining a well-fed diet.

Fish is high in safe fatty acids of omega-3. Select fish caught in the wild and in areas free from mercury, e.g., Tuna, Catfish, Halibut, Flounder, Cod, Mahi-mahi, Snapper, Trout, Salmon, and Mackerel

Shellfish - Clams, Squid, Oysters, Crab, Lobster, Mussel, Scallops

Carbohydrates

The primary carbohydrate sources in the ketogenic diet consist of vegetables. Organic vegetables are excellent choices. There is little difference between natural and organic in terms of nutritional value. The distinction is the risk of consuming vegetables with dark leafy vegetables containing the least good carbohydrate content, e.g., Spinach, Watercress, All types Cabbage, All kinds Lettuce, Kale, Brussels sprouts, Broccoli, Celery, Cucumber, Cauliflower, Bean sprouts, Radishes, Asparagus

Milk and Dairy Products

For ketogenic diets, meat and dairy products are essential. Preference is given to pure and natural products. In the case of non-fat or minimal fat, the full-fat option is also best preferred.

In the ketogenic diet, eggs are essentials. It is a major source of fats and proteins.

It is also best to include your cream in your diet. This provides more complex aromas.

Hard or soft types of cheese. It is made of carbohydrates. Bring cheeses into the daily count of carbohydrates.

Nuts

Throughout ketogenic diets, mild nut intake is tolerated. Proteins, fats, and carbohydrates can be found in nuts. The nut type should be evaluated for the overall carbohydrate, fat and protein composition and included in daily keto measurements. The best way to remove anything that can disrupt or interfere with the body's ketosis is to roast nuts and seeds.

- Mostly the nuts are offered as a snack
- Almonds, macadamias, and walnuts are good nuts to include.
- Many foods are high in omega-6 fatty acids that can cause the body to swell.
- The higher amount of carbohydrates are found in the pistachio and cashew. It's best to properly rack these

Spices

Adjustment to less carbohydrate intake may be challenging during the first few weeks of following a ketogenic diet. Those with a sweet tooth can find too much to handle for their cravings. Persons who eat high carbohydrate foods, such as pasta and processed foods may complain about bland and not so tasty foods. After some time, ketogenic diets might be dull. Spices could spice up things. To make eating somewhat more entertaining and enjoyable to the palate, new and dried spices can be added to foods and beverages.

Carbohydrate is a component of spices. Even a handful of extra spices in daily carbs and ketogenic counts should be included. Pre-made blends of seasoning typically contain added sugars. Read the labels so that the total number of carbohydrates is accurately reported.

The savor can be strengthened by sugar. Pick sea salt over table salt because there's ground dextrose in table salt. This is a sugar that in a ketogenic diet should be avoided.

Spices can also be added for the various health benefits offered not only for the spices, but also. Some of these beneficial spices include: Basil, Black pepper, Cayenne pepper, Cilantro, Cinnamon, Chili powder, Cumin, Parsley, Oregano, Sage, Rosemary, Turmeric, Thyme

Sweeteners

For curbing carbohydrates and sweets cravings, artificial sweeteners are beneficial. They help to ensure that the ketogenic diet is adhered to. Artificial sweeteners like Stevia and E-Z sweets are the best to try out. The carbohydrate count is not impaired. The fluid form was chosen when selecting sweeteners because no binders, such as dextrose or maltodextrin are applied. Some of the proposed sweeteners are as follows: Sucralose, Xylitol, Erythritol, Monk fruit

Beverages

The inadequate intake of carbohydrates affects the body diuretically. Carbohydrates draw water from them while retaining water. The reduction of carbohydrates in the diet preserves less water and excretes more. This can prevent a person from being dehydrated. It is a must to drink everyday sufficient volumes of liquids. When the body loses more fluid, there is also a greater risk of urinary tract infections and bladder pain.

Drink 8 glasses more than the maximum recommended daily consumption. Increasing hydration of your skin by adding certain forms of liquids. The normal fluid intake can also include espresso and teas. Alone coffee and tea do not affect the ketosis state greatly, but the additional substances may affect. Pick artificial sweetening agents. Or drink full cream of coffee or tea, a combination of all without sugar.

The best way to take energy smoothies and protein shakes is not to smooth bananas. The fruits contain sugar, which can interfere with ketosis. Vegetable juice also offers great drinks ideas on a ketogenic diet with the permitted vegetable forms.

8 What Are The Restricted Foods

Carbohydrates are specifically linked to ketosis induction. The body will, however, adjust to the switch in diets. Proteins and fats must, therefore, also be regulated.

Fats - In a ketogenic diet, fats are generally welcomed. During ketosis, it is the most critical energy source. Fats must provide for around 60 to 80% of daily calorie requirements. The importance of ketogenic food depends on its value. Many individuals may even use fats as 90% of the overall daily epileptic calories.

Nonetheless, when selecting the fat type there are some rules to follow.

- Avoid trans or hydrogenated fats. These are associated with an increased risk of coronary cardiovascular disease and other disorders.
- No polyunsaturated. Omega-6 fats are usually highly inflammatory, e.g., Corn oil, Soy, Cottonseed
- Avoid seed and nut-based oil because both are rich in omega-6, and can cause inflammation in the

body, e.g., Almond oil, Flaxseed oil, Sesame seed oil

- Stay away from commercial dressings for salad and mayonnaise. If unavoidable, test the carbohydrate content.

Proteins - Protein selection is very critical because, over time, it can affect the diet. Steroid and antibiotic-treated animals can cause problems for your health Choose grass-fed, organic and free-range foods. Remove hormone-fed ones, in general rBST. Nonetheless, test the number of carbohydrates, which could come from extension materials or fillers used, when choosing processed meat items. Do not use honey and sugar to treat meats.

Carbohydrates - Intake in carbohydrates is limited by the ketogenic diet primarily. The limit is dependent on the level of activity and the metabolic rate of the individual The ketogenic diet usually requires fewer than 50 to 60 grams of the net consumption of carbohydrate daily. People with a healthy metabolism and higher rates of metabolism (for example, athletes) can eat up to 100 or more grams per day in carbohydrates. Inactive people with Type 2 diabetes mellitus can consume less than 30 grams of carbohydrates a day. Tolerance and the health condition depend on it. The purpose of the ketogenic diet is also essential.

Vegetables: While vegetables are the principal sources of carbohydrate in the ketogenic diet, other sources must be prevented. Many vegetables, including peppers, tomatoes, and onions, have a high content of sugar. Many underground vegetables contain carbohydrates and are starchy.

Sweets: Stay away from the normal sweet foods because the sugars and carbs are extremely high. These are: Ice creams, Puddings, Jam (all forms, including diabetic jam), Flavored yoghurt (the artificial flavoring may contain sugar as maltodextrin or in some other form), Chocolate mix drinks (like Ovaltine, Milo, and Quik), Condensed milk, Chocolates (these include diet chocolate and other chocolate variants including lollies), Sweetened syrups and toppings, Milk flavorings, Pickles and chutneys, Biscuits (plain, with cream filling, iced or chocolate coated), Pies, Pastries, Cakes, Sauces, Bread and buns, Chewing gum (even the ones without sugar), Glace Fruit, Fruit juice, Cordials and soft drinks that contain sugar, Sweetened cough syrups, and medications, Sweetbreads.

Sugars: Sugar is a wealthy glucose source and should be discouraged. Sugar is generally known in ways, such as brown sugar, red, beaver and icing sugar. It can also be used in refined foodstuffs and pharmaceutical items.

Alcohol - Many alcoholic drinks are low in glycemic content and ideal for a ketogenic diet. Yet bear in mind that your liver tends to treat ethanol and stop producing ketones when you drink alcohol. Reduce your alcohol intake to a minimum, if you are on a Ketogenic diet to lose weight. Stick with the low sugar blenders to stop some beer and wine if you're looking for a drink.

Seed Oils - Seed oil is heavily processed and oxidized (ACA, rancid) when heated. Maize, canola oil, peanut oil, and grapefruit oil should also be avoided. These are also rich in omega-6 fatty acids that are highly inflammatory.

9 How To Start A Keto Diet

It can be daunting if you want to start a keto diet, but we all have to pick up from somewhere. The key point of implementing a keto diet is:

Restrict Carbohydrates. This is the key thing! Restrict net carbohydrates for a keto diet to less than 20 g per day. Many individuals may get away with less than 30 g. For a low-carb diet, strive for less than 50 g net carbs per day, although some modifications are between 50-100 g per day. Drop the carb limit and you are already half of the way there!

Limit protein intake. A low carbohydrate diet or low keto diet does not mean a high protein diet. Low carb in protein is normally higher than keto, but be vigilant about both. High intakes of protein can strain the kidneys, and excess protein can also be transformed into glucose. Make a daily target for your protein intake, but more than that.

Use fat as a lever. We were told to be scared of fat, but you don't have to be! The low carb and keto diets are high in fat. Protein is both our energy source and our satiety. Nevertheless, fat is a component of low carb and Keto diet, the secret to learning. Carbs and protein remain constant, with fat increasing or decreasing (pushing up or down the lever) respectively to raise or lower weight. If your goal is to lose weight, then consume enough fat to be comfortable, but once you are satisfied, no need to "Put your fats in."

Drink lots of water. In a low carb or keto diet, this is particularly important. Why is this so? The body stores the excess in the liver when you eat carbohydrates, where it is bound to water molecules. Low-carb intake depletes this glycogen, which helps you to burn fat, but it also ensures that you save less water to make dehydrated faster. Mount 16 cups to pursue a low carbohydrate diet instead of the standard guideline of eight cups a day.

Keep up the electrolytes. Sodium, potassium, and magnesium are the main electrolytes in our bodies. Due to the reduction in the amount of water you carry, a low carb (especially a keto diet) diet can flush out electrolytes and make you feel sick (called keto influenza). This is temporary, but by freeing your meat, drinking broth (particularly bone broth) and eating wetted vegetables you can prevent or remove it. Many patients may also choose to take electrolyte supplements, but a doctor who knows and supports keto/low carb diets should first be approached.

Eat only when you are hungry. Take the idea that you must eat 4-6 meals a day or snack continuously. It is not necessary to eat too often on a keto or low carb diet, which can cause loss of weight. Eat if you're hungry, but don't if you're not. It would be much easier to eat fewer carbs because this obviously suppresses the appetite.

Focus on whole foods. Although it is legally not necessary to restrict carbs or eat natural or whole foods, consuming prepared foods will not allow you to get out of cravings or to be good for your body.

Exercise. This is not needed nor recommended for a low carb diet. You will feel better, improve the health and it will happen faster if your target is weight loss!

9.1   Calculating And Hitting Your Macros For Keto

Perhaps without tracking your macronutrients, you know what you have to do to move to keto, but you are really right. Holding the macros correctly is the main part of the commencement of a ketogenic diet.

Sure, recording macros can be boring and repetitive, but it's absolutely essential during the first few weeks of a keto diet. The diet is probably contradictory to everything you've been doing before, and monitoring your macro gives guidance and helps you to troubleshoot before you stay out of it.' You can either get the proteins up or down and the fat goes up. When you come from an American standard diet, then the carbohydrates go up. You'll be able to take your fat intake to shocking levels, and your protein may fall significantly if you're from a bodybuilding diet.

A keto diet plan is a high fat and moderate-protein alternative to the macro-distribution that is limited by carbohydrates. Here's how most of the macros finally look for:

- Fats: 70-75 percent
- Carbohydrates: 5-10 percent
- Protein: 15-20 percent

Call for carbs and protein to continue your measurements and keep your carbohydrates under 50 grams daily. I just prescribe 5% calories from carbohydrates, which usually reach less than 30 grams on average. I see why people feel anxious and uncomfortable wondering 'Should I even eat a salad?' I suggest that you monitor 'net carbs', which is full carbs minus fiber. An Avocado, for example, contains 12g of carbs with 10g of fiber indicating that it has 2g of net carbs. Green leafy vegetables are also very fiber-friendly so that you can eat them about as much as you want and live under the limit

In terms of protein, it is often recommended that athletes following a ketogenic diet set protein between 0.6 and 1.0 grams per pound of lean mass - not per pound of body weight. Below is an example of how you could calculate the protein needs of a 180-pound lifter who has 15 percent body fat:

180 lbs. x 0.15 = 27 lbs. of fat

180 lbs. - 27lbs. = 153 lbs. lean mass

153 lbs. x 0.6 g = 91.8 g

153 lbs. x 1.0g = 153 g

Protein range = 92-150 g per day

You can either check or multiply your daily intake with 0.15-0.20 to measure a daily protein allowance by using our calculator if you do not know the percentage of body fat.

Why So Little Protein On Keto?

You may be cynical about a diet that needs you to minimize protein consumption by up to half if you're used to a protein intake well over the weight of your body — leave your lean body mass alone.

Protein

At first, I was terribly worried that because of the reduced intake of protein I would lose muscle capacity. On the other hand, I definitely didn't lose a muscle. How can that be? It is because of the 'protein-sparing' role of ketones. There is no need for lots of food.

What if you go too far, what happens? Simple: Tell ketosis goodbye! Many amino acids are gluconeogenic, and carbohydrates can actually be made.

In other words, it could end up with the same result as eating too many carbohydrates if your protein intake is too high. That said you can begin to play on how much protein you eat in a day until you gain additional familiarity with your personal levels of ketosis.

9.2   Living The Fat Life

The macro in the ketogenic diet that can be readily measured is fat. Once you have your carbs and protein, just satisfy your calorie requirements with fat sources for the remainder. If you want to gain some weight, add about 55 grams or 500 calories. Cut your fat consumption by 22-55 grams or 200-500 calories if you want to lose some weight.

When a ketogenic diet is adopted, most people are immediately reluctant to lather it with fat phobias.

It was extremely hard. You spend your whole life hearing stories of how obesity causes strokes or heart attacks. Immediately, every day you eat 200 grams of fat. Before you can achieve success with the keto diet, you'll have a huge psychological dimension to overcome. At first, it's like trying to persuade people a thousand years ago that the world's round and not flat anymore. But, once you begin your diet, it can be hard to get enough fat. On the menu are nuts, coconut, butter, almonds, chocolate, olive oil, and fatty meat cuts. Do not be excessive with polyunsaturated fats like maize, soybean and sunflower oil. Dieters who raise their fat consumption frequently end up in gastrointestinal distress, which brings them to the jump deck.

9.3 Defeating The "Keto Flu"

You may have heard horror stories about what athletes experience when they cut carbs or when they're talking about their keto journey. Nonetheless, the chances are that they are not in ketosis but, above all, in compliance with a well-formulated ketogenic diet. Sure, you can feel some fogginess or pain, but if you do it correctly, it doesn't have to be intense

Within a few days of cutting carbohydrate and fat elevation, the blood levels of ketone and the brain should start to use them preferentially for energy. The initial process of keto adjustment usually takes approximately four weeks, at which stage you are going to achieve maximum fat-burning improvements.

Virtually the whole keto side effects happen in the first four months, even the first 4-5 days. Experienced ketogenic dieters, such as Wittrock claim that they can be often attributed to a single cause, namely a lack of electrolytes.

Most people just jump in, feeling it is only carb-cutting and rising fat they have to do. You get 'keto flu' all of a sudden and feel tired, lethargic and experience frequent headaches. The main reason for this is the absence of the three main electrolytes: potassium, magnesium, and sodium. You will fail both mentally and physically if you are lacking in any of them. This is the main reason why people struggle in their keto diet.

So how can you get enough of these three important electrolytes? Well, supplements can be used, but you don't have to. A better solution is to change your meal schedule a little.

Salt - I encourage you to salt your food eat salty snacks and use chicken broth for sodium. Sodium production is difficult for people to understand because sodium intake is connected with water retention and fat loss. Nonetheless, it is important to substitute your missing sodium, particularly if you work out.

Meet your new best friends: avocados, vegetables, and almonds, for the other two electrolytes. Eat 1-2 avocados a day. A great source of potassium and magnesium are also green leafy vegetables.

Magnesium is also the most abundant to the fattiest nuts and seeds, such as almonds, pistachios, pecan nuts, and pumpkin seeds. Make them part of your keto diet daily, but do not be afraid to use the supplement if needed.

When you begin to feel the headaches and pains, throw a bouillon cube with a tablespoon or two of salted butter into a mug of hot water. This not only relieves some of the effects, but also provides an easy way to digest lower fat.

9.4   Keto-Friendly Supplements

As the prevalence of a ketogenic diet continues to increase, interest in health improvement continues in line with this fatty low-carb diet. Since the keto diet eliminates a set of food options, the introduction of specific nutrients is a good idea. Not to mention, certain supplements that help dietitians to reduce the difficulty of keto flu and even improve athletic performance in low-carb diet practice. Here are the perfect alternatives to a keto diet.

Magnesium

Magnesium is an energy-enhancing mineral that controls your blood sugar and supports your immune system. Research suggests that a large portion of the population has or is likely to develop a magnesium deficiency because of magnesium depleting drugs, the dependence on processed foods and other causes. With a ketogenic diet, you may have even greater magnesium requirements because many foods with an abundance of magnesium, such as beans and vegetables, are high in carbs.

That's why it might be helpful if you are on the keto diet to take 200–400 mg of magnesium per day. Magnesium supplementation may help to reduce muscle cramps, sleeping problems, and irritability–all symptoms that are typical to those who have a ketogenic diet. Magnesium glycinate, magnesium gluconate, and magnesium citrate are among the most absorbable sources of magnesium.

Incorporate these low-carb and rich-magnesium options: spinach, avocado, swiss chard, mackerel and Pumpkin seeds if you wish to raise your magnesium intake through keto-friendly meals.

MCT Oil

Medium-chain triglycerides, or MCTs, are a common addition to keto dietary foods. The metabolization of triglyceride, the most common fat in foodstuffs, is distinct from that of long chains. MCTs are broken down by the liver and can easily be used as a source of the energy for your brain and muscles in your bloodstream. Coconut oil is one of MCT's best natural sources, with about 17% of its fatty acids being MCT's and possible metabolic advantages.

Nevertheless, the use of MCT oil (made from coconut and palm oil insulation by MCTs) offers an even more intense MCT dosage and can be useful to ketogenic people following the diet.

MCT oil supplements should benefit your dietary supplements because they can easily increase your fat intake and allow you to live in ketosis. The weight loss and feelings of completeness have also been shown to be encouraged, which can benefit those who use ketogenic eating as a method of weight loss. Shaking and smoothing of MCT oil can be easily added and taken with the spoonful just to improve the fat.

A small dose of MCT oil is a great idea to start by seeing how the body reacts before the recommended doses on the supplementary container. In some cases, MCT oil can cause symptoms, such as diarrhea and vomiting.

Omega-3 Fatty Acids

The foods with Omega-3 fatty acids, including tuna and krill oil, are high in Eicosapentaenoic Acid (EPA) and Docosahexaenoic Acid (DHA), which support nutrition in a variety of ways. It has been observed that EPA and DHA reduce the risk of inflammation, cardiovascular disease, and mental decline. The west diets appear to be higher in omega-6 fatty acids and lower in omega-3 fatty acids.

This disequilibrium can cause inflammation of the skin and has been associated with a rise in many inflammatory diseases. Omega-3 supplements can be especially beneficial for ketogenesis consumers because after having a high-fat diet, they can help maintain a healthy omega-3 to omega-6 ratio. In addition, omega-3 supplements can optimize the overall health benefit of the ketogenic diet.

One research has shown that the triglycerides, leptin and inflammatory markers have reduced more than those in ketogenic dicts that have been complemented with mega-3 fatty acids from krill oil.

Choose a reputable company that offers at least 500 mg EPA/DHA in a combined 1,000 mg serving while shopping for omega-3 supplements. Individuals who use omega-3 supplements should be checked with a specialist before using them as they can improve your risk of bleeding by diluting their plasma. Use more tuna, sardines, and anchovies to improve the consumption of omega-3 fatty acids by consuming keto-friendly diets.

Vitamin D

It is critical for everyone's wellbeing to have maximum vitamin D levels, even individuals following ketogenic diets. The keto diet doesn't need to make you more likely to develop a vitamin D deficiency; however, as the lack of the vitamin D, in particular, is normal, it's a good idea to replace it. For many body functions, vitamin D is essential, including to promote the absorption of calcium, a nutrient that could be lacking from ketogenic diets, especially lactose intolerant. Vitamin D also strengthens the immune system, regulates cell growth, improves bone health and reduces body inflammation.

Because few of these essential vitamin products are good sources, most health professionals prescribe supplements of vitamin D to ensure proper consumption. A blood test may be done by your doctor to check if you are in vitamin D deficiency or help you administer an appropriate dose depending on your needs.

Digestive Enzymes

One of the biggest concerns of those who just started a ketogenic diet is that its high-fat content is hard to digest. As the keto diet can be up to 75% of fat, painful digestive symptoms, such as vomiting or diarrhea can happen if a diet is smaller than healthy. Therefore, although the ketogenic diet is the only medium in protein, it can be better than some people who also suffer gastrointestinal side effects.

A digestive enzyme mix that includes enzymes that break down fat (lipases) and protéins (proteases) can improve digestion when you have digestive problems including diarrhea, diarrhea and floating after switching to a Ketogenic diet. In addition, proteolytic enzymes, enzymes that contribute to breaking down and digesting protein, showed a reduced painful post-working, which can be a good bonus for those who like a training diet.

Exogenous Ketones

Exogenous ketones are ketones provided by an exterior source while endogenous ketones are the kind that your body produces spontaneously through a cycle named ketogenesis. Exogenous ketone additives are often used to increase blood ketone levels in those who adopt a ketogenic diet. Besides being able to help you to achieve ketosis quicker, exogenous ketone supplements were also correlated with other advantages. For instance, athletic performance, muscle regeneration rate and appetite decrease have shown to be improved. Evidence on exogenous ketones, however, is minimal, and many experts argue that keto-dieters do not need this supplement.

Furthermore, many research on exogenous ketones employed a more active type of exogenous ketone ketone ketone esters rather than ketone salts, the most common form associated in consumer-only supplements. While these supplements may be useful to some patients, further research is needed to determine their possible risks and benefits. Exogenous ketones may lead to increasing ketone levels, reduced appetite, and increased sportive efficiency. Further work is, however, needed to make these supplements further successful.

Fiber

During a keto diet, fiber supplements can assist with constipation. Fiber is the indigestible component of vegetable food and necessary for the health of the digestive system. A human can become constipated without enough fiber. Depending on your age and gender, people should get 25-31 grams of fiber per day.

There are many helpful foodstuffs containing fibers, including almonds, beans, avocado, and vegetables. On the other hand, if someone insists on fish, seafood, eggs, and dairy, the keto diet may not be filled with enough protein. Fiber supplements can help if people feel that during the keto diet they are constipated. They will look for a non-sugar-friendly formula. Drink plenty of water is also essential and helps to keep digestion moist. Taking the addition of fiber without sufficient water consumption can intensify constipation.

Greens Powder

Everyone should focus on increasing vegetable intake. The vegetables include a wide range of nutrients, minerals, and strong plant compounds to prevent inflammation, reduce your risk of infection and help your body operate optimally. While everybody who practices a keto diatribe does not actually have a shortage of vegetables, this eating plan makes it harder to consume plant food. An easy and fast way to increase your consumption rate in vegetables is to apply a greens powder to your diet. Powdered plants like spirulina, chlorella, cabbage, broccoli, wheatgrass and more are a variety of most organic powders. Green powders can be applied to juices, shakes, and smoothies, thereby increasing the safe consumption. Those who follow Ketogenic diets can also focus on adding to their meals and snacks more whole meat, low carbon vegetables. A well-balanced paste is an ideal and easy way for keto Dieters to provide a nutritional boost to their meal plan while this is not a replacement for fresh foods.

Electrolyte Supplements or Mineral-Rich Foods

It is important to focus on adding minerals via diet, particularly when you first switch to a ketogenic diet. The first weeks can be tough because the body will try to adapt to the very low consumption of carbohydrates. The change to a ketogenic diet increases the body's water loss. Potassium, sodium, and magnesium concentrations can also decline to lead to keto flu symptoms, including muscle cramps, nausea, and tiredness. Athletes who follow a keto diet may also experience more loss of water and electrolytes by sweating.

The best strategy is to add sodium via diet. It should be easy for people to salt meat or to drink on a broth made of bouillon cubes. An increase in your consumption of foods rich in potassium and magnesium can also reduce the deficiencies of these essential minerals. Dark leafy greens and pasta, avocados and sows are all keto-friendly and magnesium-friendly foods. Sodium, potassium, and magnesium supplements are also available.

Supplements to Boost Athletic Performance

The following supplements can benefit athletes seeking to increase efficiency while on a ketogenic diet:

Creatine monohydrate: Creatine monohydrate has been shown to encourage muscle gains, boost fitness efficiency and increase endurance.

Caffeine: An additional cup of green coffee or tea can improve athletic performance and energy levels, especially in athletes who newly turned to the keto diet.

Branched-Chain Amino Acids (BCAAs): BCAA supplements are found to reduce muscle soreness, muscle damage, and exercise-related fatigue.

Beta-hydroxy beta-methyl butyrate (HMB): HMB can help to reduce muscle loss and increase muscle mass particularly in those who have just begun a training and increased the strength of their training.

Beta-alanine: Amino acid beta-alanine supplements may help to avoid tiredness and muscle fatigue from taking the ketogenic diet.

10 Breakfast

10.1 Egg Cups with Bacon

Prep time: 10 minutes; Cooking time: 15 minutes; Servings: 4

Ingredients:

- ½ teaspoon paprika
- 1 tablespoon butter
- ¼ teaspoon salt
- ½ teaspoon dried dill
- 4 eggs
- 6 oz. bacon

Directions:

In the blender pot, beat the eggs. Paprika, salt, and dried dill are then added. Using the hand blender, carefully mix the egg mixture.

Then pour the butter over four ramekins.

Cut the bacon and put it in cup shape in ready-made ramekins.

Dress the egg mix with bacon in the middle of each ramekin.

Put Air fryer at 360 F.

Place the ramekins in the Air fryer and cover it.

Cook for 15 minutes.

When the time is finished, the mixture of eggs and bacon should be delicious.

Take out the egg cups and serve.

Nutrition: Calories 319, Fat 25.1, Fiber 0.1, Carbs 1.2, Protein 21.4

10.2 Eggs in Avocado Boards

Prep time: 8 minutes; Cooking time: 15 minutes; Servings: 2

Ingredients:

- 2 eggs
- 1 teaspoon butter
- ¼ teaspoon flax seeds
- ¼ teaspoon ground black pepper

- ¼ teaspoon salt

- 1 avocado, pitted

- ¼ teaspoon turmeric

Directions:

Take the shallow cup, and mix the flax seeds, turmeric, ground black pepper, and salt. Gently shake it to make homogeneous.

Cut the avocado into 2 segments, after that.

Beat the eggs in the different cups.

Sprinkle the spice mixture on the eggs.

Then gently place the eggs in the halves of the avocado.

Place the avocado boards in the air fryer.

Switch the Air fryer to 355F and then cover it.

Cook the platter for 15 minutes. After 10 minutes of cooking, open the air fryer - if you want, you can remove the texture of the eggs or keep cooking to make the eggs firm.

Serve the meal right away!

Nutrition: Calories 288, Fat 26, Fiber 6.9, Carbs 9.4, Protein 7.6

10.3 Morning Ham Hash

Prep time: 10 minutes; Cooking time: 10 minutes; Servings: 3

Ingredients:

- 1 teaspoon ground black pepper
- 1 egg
- 1 tablespoon butter
- ½ onion
- 1 teaspoon paprika
- 5 oz. Parmesan
- 10 oz. ham

Directions:

Chop the Parmesan cheese.

Cut the ham into the little strips, after that.

Peel, and dice the onion.

Beat the egg in a bowl and whisk it, using the hand whisker.

Add the butter, strips of ham, diced onion, and salt.

Sprinkle the blend with the ground black pepper and paprika after this. Then mix it up.

Heat up the air fryer to 350F.

Move the ham mixture into three ramekins and slather with shredded Parmesan cheese.

Put the ramekins in the preheated air fryer, and let it cook for 10 minutes.

When the time is up – extract the ramekins from the air fryer and mix the ham hash with the help of a fork.

Serve the meal!

Nutrition: Calories 372, Fat 23.7, Fiber 2.1, Carbs 8, Protein 33.2

10.4 Cloud Eggs

Prep time: 8 minutes; Cooking time: 4 minutes; Servings: 2

Ingredients:

- 1 teaspoon butter
- 2 eggs

Directions:

Separate the eggs and the egg yolks from the egg whites.

Then whisk the egg whites with the aid of the hand mixer until the white peaks are strong.

After that, spread the butter over the air fryer basket tray.

Heat up the air fryer to 300 F.

Get the egg white peaks medium clouds in the ready air fryer basket tray.

In the Air Fryer, position the basket tray and cook the cloud eggs for two minutes.

Take away the basket from the air Fryer after this, place the egg yolks in the middle of each egg cloud, and return the basket to the air fryer.

Cook the dish for an extra 2 minutes.

Then extract the cooked meal from the basket and serve.

Nutrition: Calories 80, Fat 6.3, Fiber 0, Carbs 0.3, Protein 5.6

10.5 Baked Bacon Egg Cups

Prep time: 10 minutes; Cooking time: 12 minutes; Servings: 2

Ingredients:

- ½ teaspoon paprika
- 1 tablespoon chives
- 2 eggs
- 3 oz. Cheddar cheese, shredded
- ¼ teaspoon salt
- ½ teaspoon cayenne pepper
- 4 oz. bacon
- ½ teaspoon butter

Directions:

Cut the bacon in small bits and sprinkle with cayenne pepper and paprika.

Use your fingertips to mix the cut bacon.

Then spread the butter on the ramekins and beat the eggs.

Add the cheese and cabbage shredded.

Then placed the cut bacon on the cabbage.

In the Air fryer basket put the ramekins and pre-heat the air fryer to 360F.

Place the fryer basket in the air fryer with the ramekins and cook for 12 minutes.

When the time is done, take the ramekins out of the air fryer and let it cool down for some minutes.

Carefully take the ramekins out of the bacon egg cups.

Nutrition: calories 553, fat 43.3, fiber 0.4, carbs 2.3, protein 37.3

10.6 Cauliflower Fritters

Prep time: 10 minutes; Cooking time: 15 minutes; Servings: 4

Ingredients:

- 1 tablespoon parsley
- ½ teaspoon ground white pepper
- 1 tablespoon almond flour
- 1 teaspoon olive oil
- 1 teaspoon salt
- 10 oz. cauliflower

- 1 tablespoon dried dill

- 1 egg

Directions:

Carefully wash the cauliflower, then cut it into the pieces.

Then put the cauliflower inside the blender and blend properly.

Beat the egg in the cauliflower mix and continue mixing for another 1 minute.

The blended cauliflower mixture should be moved into the bowl after this.

Sprinkle with almond flour, dried dill, salt, white pepper, and parsley.

Mix it thoroughly with a spoon.

Heat up the air fryer to about 355 F.

Then sprinkle olive oil on the air fryer basket tray.

Create the cauliflower mixture fritters and place them in the basket tray of the air fryer.

Cover the air fryer and allow the fritters to cook for about 8 minutes.

Flip the fritters to another side after this, and cook them for an extra 7 minutes.

Serve the fitters hot as soon as you confirm that they are cooked.

Nutrition: Calories 54, Fat 3.1, Fiber 2.1, Carbs 4.8, Protein 3.3

10.7 Egg-Meat Rolls

Prep time: 15 minutes; Cooking time: 8 minutes; Servings: 6

Ingredients:

- 1 teaspoon ground black pepper
- 1 tablespoon olive oil
- 1 teaspoon salt
- 1 teaspoon paprika
- ½ cup almond flour
- ¼ cup of water
- 1 egg
- 7 oz. ground beef

Directions:

Preheat the water before boiling starts.

Then mix the salt with the almond flour, and stir.

Include the boiling water, and gently whisk until the mix is homogenous.

Then knead the fluffy and smooth flour.

Leave the dough.

In the meantime, the ground beef should be mixed with the paprika and ground black pepper.

Mix up the mixture and move to the saucepan.

Roast the meat mixture over medium heat for 5 minutes. Stir it up regularly.

After that, beat and scramble the egg in the meat mixture.

Cook the ground beef mixture for another 4 minutes.

Roll the dough and then slice it into the 6 squares.

Place the mixture of the ground beef on every square.

Roll out the squares to make sticks for the dough.

Sprinkle with olive oil over the dough sticks.

Place the prepared dough sticks in the air-fryer basket after that.

Preheat the air fryer to 350 F and place the rolls of egg-meat in it.

Cook for eight minutes.

When you confirm that the egg-meat rolls are fully cooked - move them straight to the serving plates.

Nutrition: Calories 150, Fat 9.6, Fiber 1.2, Carbs 2.5, Protein 13

10.8 Classic Egg Rolls

Prep time: 10 minutes; Cooking time: 8 minutes; Servings: 4

Ingredients:

- 1 tablespoon olive oil
- 2 tablespoon water, boiled, hot
- 4 eggs
- 1 teaspoon chives
- 1 teaspoon paprika

- 1 teaspoon butter
- 6 tablespoon coconut flour
- ½ teaspoon salt

Directions:

Place the coconut flour in the dish.

Add hot boiled water and salt.

Combine it and knead the delicate dough.

Thereafter, allow the dough to rest.

In the meantime, break the eggs into the pan.

Add the chives and paprika.

Use a hand whisker to whisk it up.

Then throw the butter in the saucepan and preheat.

Pour the pancake-shaped egg mixture into the melted butter.

The egg pancake is then cooked on each side for 1 minute.

After that cut and chop the cooked egg pancake.

Roll the dough you have made and cut it into 4 squares.

Place the chopped eggs in the squares of the dough, and roll them in the shape of the stick.

Then rub the olive oil onto the egg rolls.

Preheat the fryer by air to 355 F.

Place the rolls of eggs into the basket and move the basket to the air fryer.

Cook for eight minutes.

The rolls will get light brown color when the time is up.

Serve hot on a plate.

Nutrition: Calories 148, Fat 10, Fiber 4.7, Carbs 8.2, Protein 7.1

10.9 Breakfast Sausages

Prep time: 15 minutes; Cooking time: 12 minutes; Servings: 6

Ingredients:

- 1 egg
- 1 teaspoon chili flakes
- 1 teaspoon ground coriander

- 1 teaspoon salt

- 1 tablespoon almond flour

- 7 oz. ground chicken

- ½ teaspoon nutmeg

- 1 teaspoon olive oil

- 7 oz. ground pork

- 1 teaspoon minced garlic

Directions:

In the bowl, mix the ground chicken with ground pork.

Beat the egg in the unique blend.

Then, mix it with a spoon.

Sprinkle the meat mixture with the chopped garlic, salt, nutmeg, almond flour, chili flakes and ground coriander after that.

Blend it together to make the ground meat texture smooth.

Preheat the air fryer to 360 F.

Give the ground-meat mixture medium sausages.

Sprinkle with the olive oil inside the basket tray air fryer.

The prepared sausages are then put in the air fryer basket and put in the air fryer.

Cook the sausages for about 6 minutes.

Turn the sausages into the second side after that and cook them for another 6 minutes.

When the time is up and the sausages are cooked – let them chill low.

Serve, and enjoy!

Nutrition: Calories 156, Fat 7.5, Fiber 0.6, Carbs 1.3, Protein 20.2

10.10 Breakfast Blackberry Muffins

Prep time: 15 minutes; Cooking time: 10 minutes; Servings: 5

Ingredients:

- 3 teaspoon stevia
- 1 teaspoon vanilla extract
- 4 tablespoon butter
- 3 oz. blackberry
- ½ teaspoon salt

- 1 teaspoon apple cider vinegar
- 6 tablespoon almond milk
- 1 teaspoon baking soda
- 1 cup almond flour

Directions:

In the mixing bowl, put the almond flour.

Add the salt, stevia and vanilla extract to the baking soda.

Then add almond milk, honey, and apple cider vinegar.

Smash the blackberries delicately and incorporate it into the almond flour mix.

Mix it carefully, using a fork, until the mass is uniform.

Place the muffin blend in a warm place for 5 minutes.

In the meantime, preheat the air fryer to 400F.

Begin planning muffin forms.

In the muffin forms, pour the dough. Full just half of all muffin forms.

After you have preheated the air fryer, put the muffling forms into the air fryer basket with the filling. Cover the fryer.

Cook the muffins for about 10 minutes.

If the time is running out, take away the muffins from the air fryer basket.

Chill it till it's warm.

Serve and enjoy them!

Nutrition: Calories 165, Fat 16.4, Fiber 1.9, Carbs 4, Protein 2

11 Main Dishes

11.1 Pandan Chicken

Prep time: 20 minutes; Cooking time: 10 minutes; Servings: 4

Ingredients

- 1 tablespoon butter
- 1 teaspoon stevia
- 1 teaspoon ground black pepper
- ¼ cup of coconut milk
- 1 tablespoon chives
- 1 teaspoon minced garlic
- 1 teaspoon chili flakes
- 1 teaspoon turmeric
- 15 oz. chicken
- 1 pandan leaf
- ½ onion, diced

Directions:

Cut the chicken into four large cubes.

In the large bowl, put the chicken cubes.

Sprinkle the chicken with the thin garlic, chili onion, stevia, black ground pepper, and turmeric. Cut the sprinkler with chilli.

Use your hands, mix the meat.

The pandan leaf should be cut into four sections.

Wrap in pandan leaf the chicken cubes.

Pour the cocoon milk into the bowl and leave for 10 minutes. With the wrapped chicken.

The air fryer is then preheated to 380 F.

In the air fryer basket, place the pandan chicken and cook the dish for 10 minutes.

When the chicken is cooked, move it to the plate and cool for at least 2-3 minutes.

Serve this meal!

Nutrition: Calories 250, Fat 12.6, Fiber 0.9, Carbs 3.1, Protein 29.9

11.2 Bacon Chicken Breast

Prep time: 15 minutes; Cooking time: 16 minutes; Servings: 4

Ingredients

- 1 tablespoon fresh lemon juice
- 1 teaspoon salt
- ½ teaspoon ground black pepper
- 2 tablespoon butter
- 1 teaspoon canola oil
- ¼ cup almond milk
- 1 teaspoon turmeric
- 1-pound chicken breast, skinless, boneless
- 4 oz. bacon, sliced
- 1 teaspoon paprika

Directions:

Beat the breast slightly.

Rub the spices, salts, ground black pepper and turmeric in the chicken breast.

Sprinkle the fresh lemon juice on the chicken breast.

Then put the butter and roll it in the center of the chicken breast.

In the sliced bacon, wrap the chicken roll and sprinkle the chicken with almond milk and canola oil.

Preheat the fryer of air to 380 F.

In the air fryer basket, put the chicken bacon and cook it for 8 minutes.

Turn the chicken breast to another side and cook for an additional eight minutes.

Don't worry if the bacon is very crunchy – it will give the chicken breast a juicy texture.

When the time is over, then transfer your bacon chicken breast to the serving plate and slice.

Nutrition: Calories 383, Fat 25.4, Fiber 0.7, Carbs 2.2, Protein 35.1

11.3 Cheese Chicken Drumsticks

Prep time: 18 minutes; Cooking time: 13 minutes; Servings: 4

Ingredients

- ½ teaspoon salt
- ½ teaspoon chili flakes
- 1 teaspoon dried rosemary
- 1 teaspoon dried oregano
- 1-pound chicken drumstick
- 6 oz. Cheddar cheese, sliced

Directions:

Sprinkle the dried oregano, rosemary, salt, and flakes of chili on the chicken drumsticks.

Carefully massage the chicken drumsticks and leave to marinate for 5 minutes.

Heat up the air fryer to 370 F.

In the air fryer tray, put the marinated chicken batters and cook for 10 minutes.

Place the chicken drumsticks on another side afterwards and cover with a sliced cheese layer.

Around the same time, heat the chicken for 3 minutes more.

The chicken drumsticks are then moved to a large serving tray.

Only serve the dish hot – the cheese should melt.

Nutrition: Calories 226, Fat 9.8, Fiber 0.3, Carbs 1, Protein 16.4

11.4 Succulent Beef Steak

Prep time: 15 minutes; Cooking time: 12 minutes; Servings: 4

Ingredients

- 1 tablespoon cream
- 1-pound beef steak
- 1 teaspoon ground ginger
- ½ teaspoon minced garlic
- 1 teaspoon lime zest
- 1 teaspoon dried oregano
- 1 tablespoon butter
- 2 tablespoons fresh orange juice

Directions:

Combine the orange juice fresh with the lime zest, minced garlic, ground ginger, butter, oregano, and sugar.

Nicely churn the mix.

Then the steak should be smoothly pounded.

Brush the beefsteak cautiously with churned orange juice and marinate for 7 minutes.

Preheat the fryer to 360 F after that.

In the air fryer basket, place the marinated beefsteak and cook the meat for 12 minutes. The meat should be prepared decently.

When the time is running out-pass the cooked meat to the pot.

Nutrition: Calories 245, Fat 10.2, Fiber 0.3, Carbs 1.7, Protein 34.6

11.5 Garlic Chicken

Prep time: 20 minutes; Cooking time: 16 minutes; Servings: 4

Ingredients

- 3 oz. fresh coriander root

- ¼ lemon, sliced

- 1 tablespoon dried parsley

- 1-pound chicken tights

- ½ teaspoon salt

- 1 teaspoon ground black pepper

- ½ teaspoon chili flakes

- 1 teaspoon olive oil

- 3 tablespoon minced garlic

Directions:

Peel and grind the new coriander.

Combine then olive oil, cinnamon, ground black pepper, flakes of candy and dried parsley with minced garlic.

Sprinkle the chicken tights and swirl the mixture.

Attach the sliced citrus fruit and root of grated coriander.

Carefully mix the chicken tights and marinate in the refrigerator for 10 minutes.

Preheat the fryer to 365 F in the meantime.

In the air fryer basket tub, place chicken tights.

Fill the chicken tights with all the remaining liquid and cook meat for 15 minutes.

Turn the chicken to a different side and boil for 1 minute more, until the time is over.

Serve the tights of the chicken hot.

Nutrition: Calories 187, Fat 11.4, Fiber 1, Carbs 3.6, Protein 20

11.6 Crunchy Chicken Skin

Prep time: 10 minutes; Cooking time: 6 minutes; Servings: 6

Ingredients

- ½ teaspoon ground black pepper
- ½ teaspoon chili flakes
- ½ teaspoon salt
- 1 teaspoon butter
- 1-pound chicken skin
- 1 teaspoon dried dill

Directions:

Sprinkle chili flakes, dried dill, ground black pepper, and salt on the chicken skin.

Mix up the chicken skin.

Apply the butter to the mixture of your chicken fat.

Use a knife, mix the chicken fat.

The air fryer would then preheat to 360 F.

In the air fryer bowl, put the prepared chicken skin.

Three minutes from each leg, cook the chicken skin. If you want the crunchy effect, cook the chicken skin more.

Move the cooked chicken skin to the paper towel and allow it to dry.

Serve the chicken skin.

Nutrition: calories 350, fat 31.4, fiber 0.1, carbs 0.2, protein 15.5

11.7 Air Fryer Pork Ribs

Prep time: 30 minutes; Cooking time: 30 minutes; Servings: 5

Ingredients

- 1 teaspoon mustard
- 16 oz. pork ribs
- 1 teaspoon sesame oil
- 1 teaspoon salt
- 1 teaspoon minced garlic
- 1 teaspoon chili flakes
- 1 tablespoon apple cider vinegar
- 1 teaspoon cayenne pepper
- 1 tablespoon paprika

Directions:

Cut the pork ribs roughly.

Sprinkle the pork ribs with minced garlic, cayenne powder, apples cider vinegar, mustard, and chili flakes.

Sesame oil and salt should then added.

Add the paprika and gently mix the pork ribs.

Place pork ribs for 20 minutes in the refrigerator.

Preheat the air fryer to 360 F afterwards.

Place the pork ribs in the basket of air fryer and cook for 15 minutes.

Turn the pork ribs to the other side and cook the meat for another 15 minutes.

Move the pork ribs to the serving dishes.

Nutrition: calories 265, fat 17.4, fiber 0.7, carbs 1.4, protein 24.5

11.8 Air fryer Beef Tongue

Prep time: 10 minutes; Cooking time: 20 minutes; Servings: 6

Ingredients

- 1 teaspoon ground black pepper
- 1 teaspoon paprika
- 1 tablespoon butter
- 4 cup of water
- 1-pound beef tongue
- 1 teaspoon salt

Directions:

Heat up the air fryer to 365 F.

Put the beef tongue in the bowl of the air fryer and add water.

Sprinkle oil, ground black pepper, and paprika with the mixture.

Cook the tongue of beef for 15 minutes.

After that, strain the beef tongue broth.

Break the tongue of beef into the strips.

Then throw the butter in the bowl and add the beef strips.

Cook the tongue strips of beef at 360 F for 5 minutes.

Move the dish to the service plate when the beef language is cooked.

Nutrition: Calories 234, Fat 18.8, Fiber 0.2, Carbs 0.4, Protein 14.7

11.9 Pork Rinds

Prep time: 10 minutes; Cooking time: 7 minutes; Servings: 8

Ingredients

- 1 teaspoon chili flakes
- ½ teaspoon salt
- ½ teaspoon ground black pepper
- 1-pound pork rinds
- 1 teaspoon olive oil

Directions:

Heat up the air fryer to 365 F.

Sprinkle the air fryer basket with the inside olive oil.

Then place the pork rinds on the tray of the fryer.

Sprinkle salt and chili flakes with pork rinds and black ground pepper.

Mix them gently. Balance them gently.

Cook the pork rinds for 7 minutes after that.

When the time is done, shake the pork carefully.

Move the platter to the broad serving plate and allow 1-2 minutes to chill.

Serve and eat!

Nutrition: Calories 329, Fat 20.8, Fiber 0, Carbs 0.1, Protein 36.5

11.10 Keto Salmon Pie

Prep time: 20 minutes; Cooking time: 30 minutes; Servings: 8

Ingredients

- 1 egg
- 1 onion, diced
- 1-pound salmon
- 1 tablespoon chives
- 1 teaspoon dried oregano
- 1 teaspoon dried dill
- 1 teaspoon butter
- ½ cup cream
- 1 ½ cup almond flour
- 1 teaspoon dried parsley
- 1 teaspoon ground paprika
- 1 tablespoon apple cider vinegar
- ½ teaspoon baking soda

Directions:

Beat and whisk the egg in the bowl.

Then incorporate the cream and start whisking for another 2 minutes. Before that apply baking soda and apple cider vinegar.

Fill the flour with almond and knead the non-sticky, smooth dough.

Cut the salmon into tiny bits.

Sprinkle dried oregano, dried dill, onion, chives, dried parsley and paprika on the chopped salmon.

Mix up the fish.

Split the dough into two parts.

Fill the parchment with the air fryer basket plate.

In the air fryer basket, tray put the first part of the dough and make the crust using the fingertips.

Put the salmon filling then.

Form the second portion of the dough and cover the salmon with the rolling pin.

Protect the edges of the slice.

Heat up the air fryer to 360F.

In the air fryer, put the air fryer basket tray and cook the pie for 15 minutes.

Reduce power to 355 F and cook the pastry for another 15 minutes.

When the pie is baked, remove from the bowl and chill low.

Slice the pastry and eat.

Nutrition: Calories 134, Fat 8.1, Fiber 1.1, Carbs 3.3, Protein 13.2

12 Side Dishes

12.1 Shirataki Noodles

Prep time: 5 minutes; Cooking time: 3 minutes; Servings: 4

Ingredients:

- 1 teaspoon salt
- 2 cups of water
- 8 oz shirataki noodles
- 1 tablespoon Italian seasoning

Directions:

Heat up the air fryer to 365 F.

Pour the water into the tank of the air fryer and preheat for 3 minutes.

Then add pasta, salt and Italian. Then add the shirataki.

Cook the shirataki noodles at the same temperature for 1 minute.

Then stretch and cook the noodles for another 2 minutes at 360 F.

When cooking the shirataki noodles - cool 1-2 minutes.

Mix up the noodles gently and serve.

Nutrition: Calories 16, Fat 1, Fiber 0, Carbs 1.4, Protein 0

12.2 Turmeric Cauliflower Rice

Prep time: 8 minutes; Cooking time: 10 minutes; Servings: 6

Ingredients:

- 1 teaspoon ground ginger
- 1 cup chicken stock
- 1-pound cauliflower
- 1 teaspoon turmeric
- 1 white onion, diced
- 3 tablespoon butter
- 1 teaspoon salt
- 1 teaspoon minced garlic

Directions:

Wash and cut the cauliflower roughly.

Then place the chopped cauliflower in the mixer and mix until the cauliflower has its rice texture.

Move the chocolate rice to the pot.

Attach the onion diced.

Then sprinkle with the cinnamon, turmeric, minced garlic and ground ginger in the vegetable mixture.

Mix it up.

Preheat fryer to 370 F.

Place the mixture of cauliflower rice there.

Add the chicken stock and butter.

Allow the cauliflower rice to cook for 10 minutes.

After the time's up, remove the chives from the fryer and drain the excess oil.

Mix it gently.

Nutrition: Calories 82, Fat 6, Fiber 2.4, Carbs 6.5, Protein 2

12.3 Taco Salad

Prep time: 10 minutes; Cooking time: 12 minutes; Servings: 8

Ingredients:

- 1 tomato
- ¼ cup heavy cream
- 1 cup lettuce
- 1 teaspoon chili pepper
- 1 teaspoon salt
- 1 teaspoon paprika
- ½ teaspoon chili flakes
- 1 teaspoon ground black pepper
- 12 oz. ground beef
- 1 teaspoon turmeric
- 8 oz. Cheddar cheese
- 1 tablespoon sesame oil

Directions:

Combine the ground beef with salt, onions, onions, chili flakes and black pepper.

With the aid of the fork, blend the ground meat mixture.

Sprinkle with the sesame oil the mixture of the ground beef and put it in the air bowl of the fryer.

Cook the ground beef for 12 minutes at 365 F. Remove it once when cooking.

Chop the tomato roughly and break the salad.

Place the vegetables in a big bowl of salad.

Break the cheese cheddar into the cubes and add them to the salad mix.

If the beef is cooked – let it cool until the room temperature is reached.

In the lettuce salad, add the ground beef.

Sprinkle the dish with the heavy cream and add two wooden spatulas.

Serve it!

Nutrition: Calories 160, Fat 13, Fiber 0.4, Carbs 1.5, Protein 9.5

12.4 Spiced Asparagus

Prep time: 9 minutes; Cooking time: 6 minutes; Servings: 6

Ingredients:

- 1 tablespoon sesame oil

- 1 tablespoon flax seeds

- 1 teaspoon salt

- 1-pound asparagus

- 1 teaspoon chili flakes

- ½ teaspoon ground white pepper

Directions:

Combine the salt, chili flakes, and ground white pepper with the sesame oil.

Churn the mix.

Heat up the fryer of air to 400 F.

In the air fryer basket tub, brush the asparagus with the sesame oil-spice mixture.

Cook asparagus for 6 minutes.

When the dish is cooked – allow for a few minutes to chill.

Nutrition: Calories 42, Fat 2.7, Fiber 2, Carbs 3.4, Protein 1.9

12.5 Zucchini Gratin

Prep time: 15 minutes; Cooking time: 13 minutes; Servings: 6

Ingredients:

- 1 teaspoon butter
- 1 teaspoon ground black pepper
- 2 zucchini
- 1 tablespoon coconut flour
- 1 tablespoon dried parsley
- 5 oz. Parmesan cheese, shredded

Directions:

In the big tub, mix dried parsley, cocoa meal, ground black pepper, and shredded cheese.

Shake it gently to make the mass homogeneous, wash and slice the zucchini.

Then cut the zucchini into squares.

Place the butter in the air fryer basket bowl and placed the zucchini squares.

Preheat the air fryer to 400 F.

Sprinkle with the dried parsley mixture the zucchini squares.

Cook the zucchini for 13 minutes.

When the turkey gratin is baked, the surface is light orange.

Nutrition: Calories 98, Fat 6, Fiber 1.3, Carbs 4.2, Protein 8.6

12.6 Winter Squash Spaghetti

Prep time: 10 minutes; Cooking time: 10 minutes; Servings: 8

Ingredients:

- 1 teaspoon ground black pepper
- 1 teaspoon butter
- 1-pound winter squash
- 1 teaspoon salt
- 4 tablespoons heavy cream
- 1 cup chicken stock

Directions:

Peel the squash of winter and grate it for spaghetti.

Heat up the air fryer to 400 F.

Into the air fryer basket tray, put the winter squash spaghetti.

Sprinkle with salt and chicken stock.

Apply the black pepper to the ground and cook for 10 minutes.

When the time is done, push out of the winter squash spaghetti excess oil.

Then apply the heavy cream and butter and stir.

Serve the side dish right away.

Nutrition: Calories 55, Fat 3.4, Fiber 0.9, Carbs 6.4, Protein 0.7

12.7 Kale Mash

Prep time: 10 minutes; Cooking time: 12 minutes; Servings: 7

Ingredients:

- 1 teaspoon ground black pepper
- 1 white onion, diced

- 1 teaspoon salt
- 1 cup heavy cream
- 1-pound Italian dark leaf kale
- 7 oz. Parmesan, shredded
- 1 teaspoon butter

Directions:

Chop the kale cautiously and put it in the air fryer basket tray.

Sprinkle with salt, butter, black ground pepper, diced onion, and heavy cream on the chopped kale.

Heat up the air fryer for 225F.

Cook the kale twelve minutes.

When the time is done, carefully mix the kale mash to make it homogeneous.

Serve and eat the kale mash!

Nutrition: Calories 180, Fat 13.2, Fiber 1.7, Carbs 6.8, Protein 10.9

12.8 Stewed Celery Stalk

Prep time: 10 minutes; Cooking time: 8 minutes; Servings: 6

Ingredients:

- 2 tablespoons heavy cream
- 1 teaspoon salt
- 1 white onion, sliced
- 1 cup chicken stock
- 1-pound celery stalk
- 1 tablespoon butter
- 1 tablespoon paprika

Directions:

Chop the stalk of celery roughly.

Add the chicken stock and the sliced onion to the air fryer basket plate.

Heat up the air fryer to 400 F.

Fry the onion for 4 minutes.

Subsequently, raising the heat to 365 F.

Add salt, celery chopped stalk, paprika, butter, and heavy cream.

Mix the mixture of vegetables.

Cook the celery for another 8 minutes.

The celery stalk will be very tender when the time is over.

Cool the side dish to the temperature of the room.

Serve it!

Nutrition: Calories 59, Fat 4.2, Fiber 2, Carbs 4.9, Protein 1.1

12.9 White Mushrooms With Spicy Cream

Prep time: 10 minutes; Cooking time: 12 minutes; Servings: 4

Ingredients:

- 1 onion, sliced
- 1 cup cream
- 1 teaspoon olive oil
- 1 teaspoon ground red pepper
- 9 oz. white mushrooms

- 1 teaspoon garlic, sliced
- 1 teaspoon butter
- 1 teaspoon chili flakes

Directions:

Chop the white mushrooms.

Sprinkle chili flakes and the ground red pepper on the white mushrooms.

Mix up the mix.

Heat up the air fryer to 400 F afterwards.

In the air fryer basket plate, add the olive oil.

Then add the champagne and cook the vegetables for 5 minutes.

Attach the sliced onion, milk, butter, sliced garlic and spatula to mix the mushroom gently.

Cook the dish at 365 F for 7 minutes.

Once the time is done – carefully remove the side dish.

Serve it warm.

Nutrition: Calories 84, Fat 2.9, Fiber 1.4, Carbs 7, Protein 2.9

12.10 Eggplant Stew

Prep time: 10 minutes; Cooking time: 13 minutes; Servings: 7

Ingredients:

- 1 green pepper
- 1 teaspoon dried parsley
- 1 cup chicken stock
- 2 garlic cloves, peeled
- 1 teaspoon turmeric
- 1 teaspoon paprika
- ½ cup heavy cream
- 1 eggplant
- 1 teaspoon dried dill
- 1 zucchini
- 1 onion
- 1 teaspoon kosher salt

Directions:

Divide the eggplants and the zucchini into the cubes.

Then sprinkle dried psalm, dried dill, peppers, and turmeric on the vegetables.

Chop the cloves of garlic.

Then chop onion and pepper orange.

Heat up the air fryer to 390 F.

Put in the air fryer the chicken stock and add the eggplants.

Cook the eggplants for 2 minutes.

Add the sliced onion and the green pepper afterwards.

Then apply the cloves and heavy cream of the chopped garlic.

Cook the stew at the same temperature for 11 minutes more.

Transfer to the serving plates the cooked side dish.

Serve the hot meal.

Nutrition: Calories 65, Fat 3.6, Fiber 3.5, Carbs 8.1, Protein 1.7

13 Snacks and Appetizers

13.1 Cauliflower Crispy Florets

Prep time: 15 minutes; Cooking time: 16 minutes; Servings: 8

Ingredients:

- 1 teaspoon salt
- ½ teaspoon ground black pepper
- 1 teaspoon oregano
- 1 teaspoon turmeric
- 18 oz. cauliflower
- 1 egg
- 2 tablespoons almond flour
- 1 cup heavy cream
- ½ tablespoon olive oil

Directions:

Wash and break the cauliflower into medium florets.

Beat the egg in the large bowl and whisk it afterwards.

Add cinnamon, black ground pepper, turmeric, almond meal, and oregano.

Whisk the mixture until the batter is smooth.

Coat the flower with the heavy cream batter.

Preheat the fryer with air to 360 F.

Put the coated cauliflower in the basket bowl of the air fryer.

Cook vegetables 12 minutes. Prepare them.

Following that, raise the temperature to 390 F and cook the snack for a further 4 minutes.

Chill the flowers of the cooked cauliflower.

Serve it!

Nutrition: Calories 125, Fat 10.6, Fiber 2.5, Carbs 5.7, Protein 3.8

13.2 Scotch Eggs

Prep time: 15 minutes; Cooking time: 13 minutes; Servings: 3

Ingredients:

- 1 egg
- 16 oz. ground beef
- ½ cup coconut flour
- 1 teaspoon turmeric
- 1 teaspoon salt
- 1 teaspoon ground black pepper
- 3 eggs, boiled
- 1 teaspoon olive oil

Directions:

Beat and whisk the egg in the tub.

Peel the boiled eggs next.

Combine salt, ground black pepper and turmeric with ground beef.

Mix up the mix.

Create 3 balls from the mixture of ground beef and bring in boiled eggs for small meatballs.

Then dip the meatballs into the egg whisk.

Then coat the meatballs generously in the coconut flour.

Heat up air fryer to 370 F.

Place the eggs in the scotch and spray with the olive oil.

Cook the meat for 10 minutes.

Boost the temperature to 380 F and cook the dish for another 3 minutes.

Cool the scotch eggs when cooked for a total of 2-3 minutes.

Nutrition: Calories 318, Fat 12.7, Fiber 8.3, Carbs 14.5, Protein 35.3

13.3 Eggplants Circles

Prep time: 15 minutes; Cooking time: 8 minutes; Servings: 7

Ingredients:

- 1 teaspoon ground turmeric
- 2 eggplants 1 teaspoon minced garlic
- ½ teaspoon salt
- 1 tablespoon canola oil
- 1 teaspoon dried rosemary

Directions:

Carefully wash the eggplants and cut them into thick circles.

Then combine in the bowl canola oil, hairy garlic, salt, earth turmeric, and dry rosemary.

Churn the mix.

Before that, brush the olive mixture around any eggplant.

Heat up the air fryer to 400 F.

In the air fryer rack, put the prepared eggplants around and cook for 5 minutes.

Flip the eggplant circles to another hand and cook for another 3 minutes.

If the eggplants are soft and gold-fried – they are finished.

Let them chill until the temperature of the room.

Serve the food!

Nutrition: Calories 59, Fat 2.3, Fiber 5.7, Carbs 9.7, Protein 1.6

13.4 Onion Circles

Prep time: 15 minutes; Cooking time: 8 minutes; Servings: 10

Ingredients:

- 1 egg
- 1/3 cup heavy cream
- 1/3 cup almond flour
- ½ teaspoon paprika
- ½ teaspoon ground black pepper
- 2 white onions
- ½ teaspoon salt
- ½ cup coconut flour
- 1 tablespoon olive oil

Directions:

Peel and slice the white onions roughly.

Segregate the sliced onions into the circles.

Beat and whisk the egg.

Sprinkle paprika, butter, black ground pepper and heavy cream on the whisked egg.

Whisk it back to homogeneity.

Preheat the air fryer to 360 F.

Layer the onion rings in the almond meal or dip the onion circles into the whisked egg mixture afterwards.

Coat the onion circles in the cocoa powder.

Spray the olive oil in the air fryer basket bowl and place the onion circles in it.

Cook the circles of onion for 8 minutes.

When the snack is cooked, let it cool.

Nutrition: calories 88, fat 5.7, fiber 3.3, carbs 7.1, protein 2.5

13.5 Zucchini Fritters

Prep time: 10 minutes; Cooking time: 10 minutes; Servings: 7

Ingredients:

- ½ teaspoon salt
- ½ tablespoon paprika
- 4 tablespoons coconut flour

- 1 zucchini, grated
- ¼ onion, grated
- ½ teaspoon chili flakes
- 1 egg
- 1 teaspoon butter

Directions:

In a large mixing bowl, place the grated zucchini.

Beat the egg in the zucchini.

Add coconut flour, salt, tomatoes, onion grated, and flakes of chili.

Carefully blend the mixture.

Heat up the air fryer to 365 F.

In the air fryer basket pot, melt the butter.

Then make the tiny fritters with the spoon and bring in the melted butter.

Cook the fritters from each side for 5 minutes.

Chill them well when the fritters are fried.

Nutrition: Calories 38, Fat 1.7, Fiber 2.3, Carbs 4.5, Protein 1.8

13.6 Chicken Bites

Prep time: 15 minutes; Cooking time: 15 minutes; Servings: 8

Ingredients:

- 1 teaspoon turmeric
- 2 tablespoons almond flour
- 1-pound chicken fillet
- 1 teaspoon paprika
- ½ teaspoon curry powder
- ½ cup heavy cream
- 1 teaspoon chili flakes
- 1 teaspoon olive oil

Directions:

Chop the fillet into 8 cubes.

Place the cubes of the chicken in the large cup.

Sprinkle beef, turmeric, paprika and curry powder on the chili flakes.

Mix meat with your hand.

In the separate dish, add the heavy cream and almond flour.

Whisk it properly.

Heat up the air fryer to 365 F.

In the air fryer rack, place the chicken cubes and sprinkle with the olive oil.

Heat up for 15 minutes.

Chill them well when the chicken bites are fried.

Nutrition: calories 151, fat 8.5, fiber 0.4, carbs 1, protein 17

13.7 Air Fryer Meatballs

Prep time: 10 minutes; Cooking time: 13 minutes; Servings: 7

Ingredients:

- 1 tablespoon butter
- ¼ teaspoon chili flakes
- 1 teaspoon curry paste
- 1 tablespoon tomato puree
- 1 teaspoon salt

- ½ teaspoon ground coriander
- 1 egg
- 1-pound ground beef
- ½ white onion, grated

Directions:

In the bowl, beat the egg.

Add curry paste, coriander, salt, grated onion and flakes of chili.

Mix the mixture together to absorb the curry paste.

Then add the ground beef and carefully stir until homogeneous.

Then heat up the air fryer to 366F.

Create seven small meatballs from the mixture of ground beef.

Put the meatballs then in the tank of the air fryer.

Add tomato puree and butter.

Boil the meatballs for 16 minutes.

After 7 minutes of cooking, stir the meatballs.

Transfer to the serving plate when the meatballs are ready.

Nutrition: Calories 153, Fat 6.8, Fiber 0.2, Carbs 1.2, Protein 20.6

13.8 Easy Cooked Chicken Wings

Prep time: 15 minutes; Cooking time: 12 minutes; Servings: 5

Ingredients:

- 1 teaspoon dried oregano
- 1 tablespoon olive oil
- 1-pound chicken wings
- 1 teaspoon paprika
- 1 teaspoon stevia extract
- 1 teaspoon salt

Directions:

Mix and stir in the bowl the oil, the paprika, and the dried oregano.

Slather the chicken wings with the seasoning mixture afterwards.

Sprinkle the stevia powder on the chicken wings.

Heat up the air fryer to 400 F.

In the air fryer rack, position the prepared chicken wings and douse with the olive oil.

Cook the meat for 12 minutes afterwards.

Put them on the paper towel when the chicken wings are fried.

And serve.

Nutrition: Calories 199, Fat 9.6, Fiber 0.3, Carbs 0.4, Protein 26.3

13.9 Keto French Fries

Prep time: 10 minutes; Cooking time: 15 minutes; Servings: 6

Ingredients:

- ¼ teaspoon ground white pepper
- ¼ teaspoon salt
- 1 teaspoon paprika
- 2 carrots
- 1 tablespoon olive oil

Directions:

Peel and cut the carrot into slices.

Cover with the parchment of the air fryer basket tray and put the carrot strips there.

Sprinkle with the ground white pepper, paprika and salt on the carrot strings.

Spray the olive oil on the carrot strings.

Heat up the air fryer to 365 F.

Cook the fried carrot for 15 minutes. The period depends on the thickness of the carrot strings, less or more.

Then pass the fries to the dish and chill them.

Nutrition: Calories 30, Fat 2.4, Fiber 0.7, Carbs 2.3, Protein 0.2

13.10 Eggplant Bites With Parmesan

Prep time: 8 minutes; Cooking time: 14 minutes; Servings: 4

Ingredients:

- ¼ teaspoon salt

- ½ teaspoon turmeric

- 4 oz. Parmesan, sliced

- 1 eggplant

- 1 teaspoon olive oil

Directions:

Split the eggplants into four pieces.

Slather the bites of the eggplant with turmeric, salt and blend well.

Heat up the air fryer to 400 F afterwards.

In the air fryer bowl, put the eggplants pieces and spray with olive oil.

Steam the eggplant pieces for 13 minutes after that.

Then coat the bites of the eggplant with the Parmesan sliced.

Cook the dish for another 1 minute.

Then pass the bites of the eggplant to the serving plate and chill until the cheese has become firm.

Serve!

Nutrition: Calories 131, Fat 7.5, Fiber 4.1, Carbs 7.9, Protein 10.3

14 Desserts

14.1 Peanut Butter Cookies

Prep time: 15 minutes; Cooking time: 10 minutes; Servings: 8

Ingredients:

- 8 tablespoon peanut butter
- 1 egg
- ¼ teaspoon salt
- 4 tablespoon erythritol

Directions:

Take a large bowl and pour Erythritol into it.

Add salt and peanut butter.

Then break the egg into the bowl with the mixture of peanut butter.

Mix the dough until it's homogeneous and smooth.

Then roll the dough using the rolling pin.

Create the rounds with the cutter's support.

Then make the cross in each cookie with the aid of a fork.

Heat up an air fryer to 360 F.

Place the cookies in the air fryer basket.

Cook for 10 minutes.

If cookies are baked, let them cool down.

Serve the cookies.

Nutrition: calories 102, fat 8.6, fiber 1, carbs 10.7, protein 4.7

14.2 Chia Seeds Crackers

Prep time: 15 minutes; Cooking time: 4 minutes; Servings: 8

Ingredients:

- ½ teaspoon dried rosemary
- ½ teaspoon ground ginger
- 1 oz. psyllium husk powder
- 1 teaspoon olive oil
- 1 teaspoon onion powder
- 5 tablespoon chia seeds

- 2 oz. Cheddar cheese, shredded
- ½ cup of water
- 1 teaspoon paprika

Directions:

Combine chia seeds, husk and onion powder with water.

Add peppers, dried rosemary, and ginger.

Shred Cheddar cheese and then add it to the mixture of chia seeds.

Mix up the mix to make the dough smooth. The paste should be very elastic.

Then roll the dough and use the cutter to make the medium crackers. The crackers tend to be thin.

Heat up the air fryer to 360 F.

Place the chia seeds crackers in the air fryer tray.

Four minutes cook the crackers.

Then cool the crackers and eat.

Nutrition: Calories 109, Fat 6.8, Fiber 7.2, Carbs 9, Protein 3.9

14.3 Flax Seed Crackers

Prep time: 20 minutes; Cooking time: 5 minutes; Servings:
6

Ingredients:

- ¼ teaspoon salt
- 1 teaspoon ground cinnamon
- ½ teaspoon baking soda
- 2 tablespoon swerve
- 3 oz. hot water
- 1 teaspoon apple cider vinegar
- 1 tablespoon olive oil
- 1 egg
- 8 tablespoon coconut flour
- 1 tablespoon coconut flakes
- 5 tablespoon flax seeds

Directions:

Place the flax seeds in the mixer and incorporate them into
the flour form.

Combine the seeds of flax with cocoa powder, cocoa
flakes, salt, and ground cinnamon.

In the bowl, mix baking soda and apple cider vinegar and extract them.

In the flaxseed mixture, substitute the baking soda mixture.

Delete it carefully.

Apply olive oil and hot water.

Gently whisk it and apply to swerve.

Then smash the egg in the bowl and remove it until it is a little homogeneous.

Knead the cracker dough with the fingertips afterwards.

Use more flour of almond if the dough sticks to your hands.

Then roll the cracker dough using the rolling pin.

Split the dough into the intermediate crackers.

Heat up the air fryer to 365 F.

In the air fryer basket put the crackers and cook 5 minutes.

Shake the crackers to protect against overcooking during cooking.

Let the cooked crackers cool down.

Nutrition: Calories 105, Fat 6.2, Fiber 5.9, Carbs 8.8, Protein 3.4

14.4 Sweet Fat Bombs

Prep time: 25 minutes; Cooking time: 7 minutes; Servings: 12

Ingredients:

- 3 eggs
- 1 teaspoon lime zest
- 1 teaspoon stevia extract
- 8 tablespoon fresh lemon juice
- 6 tablespoon peanut butter
- 5 tablespoon swerve
- ¼ teaspoon salt
- ½ teaspoon vanilla extract
- 2 tablespoon coconut oil
- 6 tablespoon erythritol

Directions:

Burn the peanut butter and mix with the swerve.

Then add extract of vanilla, salt, and erythritol.

Whisk the mix.

Take the truffles and place the mixture of peanut butter there.

Freeze the peanut mixture.

Heat up the air fryer to 350 F.

In the mug, add stevia extract, fresh lemon juice, lime zest, and cocoa oil.

Whisk it well.

Pour in the air fryer basket the fresh lemon mixture and cook it for 5 minutes.

Stir up every 2 minutes.

Crack the eggs and mix them with the help of the hand mixer in the lemon mixture.

If the curd is soft, cook for 2 minutes at 365 F.

Then extract and cool the cooked curd mixture.

In the pastry container, put the cooked curd mixture.

Take from the freezer the truffle.

Fill the truffles with a mixture of curds and keep the bomb cold.

Nutrition: Calories 231, Fat 24.3, Fiber 0.5, Carbs 10.3, Protein 3.5

14.5 Poppy Seeds Balls

Prep time: 20 minutes; Cooking time: 8 minutes; Servings: 11

Ingredients:

- ½ teaspoon baking powder
- ½ teaspoon apple cider vinegar
- 4 tablespoon poppy seeds
- 3 tablespoon stevia extract
- ¼ teaspoon salt
- ½ teaspoon ground cinnamon
- ½ cup heavy cream
- 1 cup coconut flour
- ¼ teaspoon ground ginger
- 1 teaspoon butter

Directions:

In the cup, combine the coconut flour, salt, cinnamon, coconut seeds, ground ginger, and baking powder.

Gently melt the butter and add to the dried mixture.

Add apple cider vinegar and stevia extract after that.

Knead the fluffy, but strong dough with the heavy cream.

Cut the log out of the prepared dough into 11 balls.

Heat up the air fryer to 365 F then.

Place balls of cotton seeds in the air fryer bowl.

Three minutes cook the wings.

Shake them little after that and cook for another five minutes.

Verify that the balls are cooked using the toothpick.

The balls can be adjusted with the size of the cotton balls.

Warm the cotton balls and place them in the paper bag or wrap them with the towel.

Nutrition: Calories 83, Fat 4.9, Fiber 4.8, Carbs 8.4, Protein 2.1

14.6 Keto Cheesecake

Prep time: 25 minutes; Cooking time: 16; Servings: 6

Ingredients:

- ½ teaspoon vanilla extract
- 2 tablespoon swerve
- 2 eggs
- ¼ teaspoon ground cinnamon
- 6 tablespoon butter, soft 1 cup cream cheese
- ½ cup almonds, sliced
- 1 tablespoon stevia extract 1 teaspoon lemon zest

Directions:

Incorporate the sliced almonds with the extract of butter, stevia, and vanilla.

Mix up the mix – cook the crust of the cheesecake.

Fill with the parchment the air fryer plate.

Place the cheesecake almond crust on the air fryer plate.

Then add swerve, ground cinnamon, citrus fruit, and cream cheese together.

Crack the eggs and mix with the side blender.

This is cooked when the mass is moist and fluffy.

Pour the mixture of cream cheese over the almond crust.

Heat up the air fryer to 310 F.

Heat up the cheesecake for about 16 minutes.

When baked, chill the cheesecake for at least 2 hours.

Cut into bits then serve.

Nutrition: Calories 307, Fat 30.4, Fiber 1.1, Carbs 3.7, Protein 6.6

14.7 Coconut Cookies

Prep time: 15 minutes; Cooking time: 10 minutes; Servings: 20

Ingredients:

- 2 teaspoon stevia extract
- 1 tablespoon coconut flakes
- 2 eggs
- ¼ teaspoon ground ginger
- 3 tablespoon coconut milk

- 1/3 cup coconut flour
- ¼ teaspoon ground cinnamon
- 3 tablespoon butter
- ¼ teaspoon salt
- ½ teaspoon vanilla extract

Directions:

Sift and put the coconut flour in the pot.

Remove flakes of coconut, butter, ginger, cinnamon ground, and vanilla extract.

Apply stevia extract after that.

Crack the eggs into the individual bowl and whisk them using a hand whisker.

Then add in the cocoon flour the whisked egg mixture.

Remove butter and milk for cocoa.

Combine it with the fork support.

If the cookie's dough is ready, make the medium balls.

Slowly and carefully flatten it.

Heat up the air fryer to 365 F.

Cover the parchment with the air fryer bowl and through the flattened cocoon balls there.

Heat up the cookies for 10 minutes.

Once the cookies are baked, the edges are light brown.

Chill and eat the cookies!

Nutrition: Calories 36, Fat 3, Fiber 0.9, Carbs 1.6, Protein 0.9

14.8 Pecan Bars

Prep time: 18 minutes; Cooking time: 23 minutes; Servings: 8

Ingredients:

- ½ teaspoon baking powder
- 1 teaspoon vanilla extract
- 2 tablespoon butter
- ½ teaspoon apple cider vinegar
- ¼ cup hot water
- ¼ teaspoon salt
- 3 tablespoon stevia extract
- ½ teaspoon sesame oil

- 1 cup almond flour
- 4 tablespoon pecans, crushed

Directions:

Heat up the butter to warm, but not liquid.

Then mix the soft butter with the meal of almond.

Then apply flour, stevia extract, vanilla extract, sugar, baking powder and vinegar of apple cider.

Sprinkle with sesame oil the almond flour mix and knead the homogeneous dough.

Then add the broken pecans and knead the dough for another 2 minutes.

Heat up the air fryer to 350 F.

Place the almond flour dough over the air fryer tray with the parchment.

Flatten to make the surface smooth.

Fill the parchment with it and cook for 20 minutes.

Replace the cover and cook the dish for another 3 minutes.

Chill the pecan dish and cut into 8 bars when the time is over.

Serve it!

Nutrition: Calories 157, Fat 14.3, Fiber 2.2, Carbs 4.1, Protein 3.7

14.9 Macadamia Nuts Brownies

Prep time: 15 minutes; Cooking time: 25 minutes; Servings: 12

Ingredients:

- 4 oz. dark chocolate, melted
- 1 cup coconut flour
- ½ teaspoon baking powder
- 3 tablespoon swerve
- 3 tablespoon butter, melted
- 2 eggs
- 1/3 cup macadamia nuts, crushed
- 1 teaspoon fresh lemon juice

Directions:

Beat and combine the eggs in a mixer bowl.

Apply melted butter and mix the mixture for another 2 minutes.

Add fresh lemon juice, melted dark chocolate, coconut flour, baking powder and swerve.

Use the silicone spatula to blend it.

Then add the split macadamia nuts and blend well.

The air fryer is then heated up to 355 F.

In the air fryer basket plate, add the brownie dough and bake for 25 minutes.

Baked brownies are meant to be fluffy, but well baked.

Break the brownies into twelve parts.

Nutrition: Calories 155, Fat 10.2, Fiber 4.6, Carbs 13.5, Protein 3.3

14.10 Coconut-Sunflower Bars

Prep time: 15 minutes; Cooking time: 16 minutes; Servings: 8

Ingredients:

- 2 tablespoon butter

- ½ cup almond flour

- 2 tablespoon coconut milk

- ¼ teaspoon salt

- 2 tablespoon stevia extract

- 2 tablespoon sunflower seeds

- 1 tablespoon coconut flakes

- 1 egg

Directions:

Crush and combine the sunflower seeds with the cocoon flakes.

Then add the salt and almond flour.

Mix the dried ingredients cautiously.

Add the egg in the blend.

Add stevia extract, butter, and coconut milk after that.

Mix with the spatula or hand mixer.

Heat up the air fryer to 355 F.

Through the air, the fryer tray pour the cocoon mixture and cook for 16 minutes.

If the mixture is too chunky – cook for 2-3 minutes longer.

Chill the cooked mixture properly.

Cut it into eight tiny bars.

Nutrition: Calories 90, Fat 8.2, Fiber 1, Carbs 2, Protein 2.5

15 Conclusion

The ketogenic diet is not only the best way to lose weight, but also to keep the body in shape. There are other advantages of this diet, such as the normalization of appetite, regulation of blood pressure and cholesterol levels.

Often, the keto diet will preserve the normal state of the human body during epilepsy. Such concern as acne can be also addressed while following such an eating lifestyle. You will note that some people are using a keto diet as a lifestyle. Otherwise, it could be harmful and could affect your health. There is a doctor's advice to start the diet for 7 days; after that, you can leave a small distance. If you change all your diet quickly, the body will have a shock, and you won't have the intended effect.

This book will help you understand how to prepare keto dishes easily and quickly. The unique, tasty and simple recipes that don't need special ingredients will make your breakfast, dinner, lunch, and even snack delicious. You can be assured that the air fryer recipes in this guide can turn your creativity about diet and food. Try the air fryer keto dishes, and you're going to give your family and friends the best holiday!